MULTI-SPECIES DEMENTIA STUDIES

Towards an Interdisciplinary Approach

Edited by
Nicholas Jenkins, Anna Jack-Waugh
and Louise Ritchie

First published in Great Britain in 2025 by

Policy Press, an imprint of
Bristol University Press
University of Bristol
1–9 Old Park Hill
Bristol
BS2 8BB
UK
t: +44 (0)117 374 6645
e: bup-info@bristol.ac.uk

Details of international sales and distribution partners are available at policy.bristoluniversitypress.co.uk

British Library Cataloguing in Publication Data
A catalogue record for this book is available from the British Library

ISBN 978-1-4473-6879-3 hardcover
ISBN 978-1-4473-6881-6 ePub
ISBN 978-1-4473-6882-3 ePdf

Cover design: Robin Hawes
Front cover image: Stocksy/Cosma Andrei
Bristol University Press and Policy Press use environmentally responsible print partners.
Printed and bound in Great Britain by CPI Group (UK) Ltd, Croydon, CR0 4YY

FSC
www.fsc.org
MIX
Paper | Supporting responsible forestry
FSC® C013604

For Henry Rankin

Contents

List of figures and tables

Figures

Table

Notes on contributors

Vanessa Ashall is a European Veterinary Specialist in Animal Welfare Science, Ethics and Law, Wellcome Trust Senior Research Fellow and Co-Director of the Science and Technology Studies Unit (SATSU), University of York. Vanessa's research examines the role of animals within our understanding of health and medicine and her current project explores the concept of the 'Good Death' across species and professional boundaries.

Jayne Beselt was Research Coordinator at the Brenda Strafford Centre on Aging at the University of Calgary from July 2021 to December 2022. Her research interests include understanding ways marginalised groups within the older adult population who are at increased risk of social exclusion and isolation experience social support and community through physical activity.

Anne Crilly is an immunologist and Lecturer in the School of Health and Life Sciences, University of the West of Scotland. Her research is focused on understanding the cellular and molecular processes which drive inflammation in chronic disease, and in the absence of infection, this is often referred to as a 'sterile inflammation'. Improved knowledge around dysregulated mechanisms which drive inflammation in chronic disease, with identification of novel targets to inform future drug discovery, are key research objectives for her. Her work has resulted in over 50 peer-reviewed papers which can be viewed here: https://research-portal.uws.ac.uk/en/persons/anne-crilly.

Gail Davies is Professor in Human Geography at the University of Exeter (UK). Her research charts the changing geographies of biomedical research and seeks to facilitate engagement between differently situated knowledges in science, technology and health. She was Co-Principal Investigator on the Animal Research Nexus Programme (2017–2023) and chaired the UK review of Harm-Benefit Analysis in her role on the UK Animals in Science Committee (2013–2019). She has published widely on the social aspects of laboratory animal research and collaborative social science methods, and is lead editor of the forthcoming book on *Researching Animal Research* (Manchester University Press, 2024).

Richard Gorman is Research Fellow in Bioethics at Brighton and Sussex Medical School, following work on the Animal Research Nexus Programme at the University of Exeter. Richard's research is interested in the social and ethical implications of different healthcare practices, and aims to be responsive to stakeholder interests, engage different publics and contribute to addressing complex policy issues. Richard has published extensively in human geography on topics related to multi-species health and wellbeing, including care farming, patient involvement and education, and the alternatives to animal research in endotoxin testing.

Fiona L. Henriquez is Professor of Parasitology and Associate Dean (Research and Innovation) in the School of Health and Life Sciences, University of the West of Scotland. Fiona's expertise is parasitology/protistology and host–pathogen interactions. She leads on research projects looking at the molecular and biochemical parasitology of protists, including *Acanthamoeba* and *Neoparamoeba, Toxoplasma gondii* and host immune response. Fiona is also interested in the interplay between the immune system and central nervous system and the impact of infection on this. Her research has resulted in over 95 peer reviewed papers which can be viewed here: https://research-portal.uws.ac.uk/en/persons/fiona-henriquez-mui.

Jennifer Hewson is Associate Professor in the Faculty of Social Work, University of Calgary. Dr Hewson is a social gerontologist with a focus on age-friendly communities, particularly older adults and social participation, support and inclusion. She is also involved in research and writing related to the relationship between older adults and companion animals and the use of animatronics in care facilities.

David B. Hogan is Professor in the Cumming School of Medicine, University of Calgary. As a specialist in geriatric medicine, his research interests have focused on the assessment and care of older adults. This would include looking at ways that technology can be used to improve the quality of life of older residents living in continuing care facilities. He has published extensively on these topics with over 365 peer-reviewed journal articles.

Anna Jack-Waugh is a mental health nurse and Senior Lecturer in Dementia at the Alzheimer Scotland Centre for Policy and Practice at the University of the West of Scotland. She leads on developing interprofessional education through research and practice for all health and social care staff working with people with dementia. Anna has been involved in projects on advanced dementia across Europe and collaborated with colleagues in India and Canada to learn from Scotland's National Dementia Champions on an international stage. In addition, Anna teaches and leads the integration of dementia education in undergraduate and postgraduate Nursing and Paramedic programmes at the University of the West of Scotland. Her work has resulted in over 30 research outputs on dementia education for all.

Nicholas Jenkins is Professor of Interdisciplinary Social Science at the University of the West of Scotland and co-founder of the Multi-Species

Dementia International Research Network. He has published on the lived experience of a range of chronic health conditions within both social science and clinical journals. Since 2014, his research has focused on the application of posthumanist and multi-species theorising in dementia.

Richard Milne is an interdisciplinary social scientist at the Kavli Centre for Ethics, Science and the Public at the University of Cambridge and Wellcome Connecting Science. His research explores ways to bring scientists and publics together around the social and ethical questions associated with emerging science and technology, most recently in the context of genomics and biodata. Richard has published widely in social science, clinical and scientific journals on the sociology of food and pharming, genomics and health data, and the ethical challenges associated with the development of new approaches to the early detection and prediction of Alzheimer's disease dementia.

Elizabeth Peel is Professor of Communication and Social Interaction at Loughborough University and Fellow of the British Psychological Society. She conducted the British Academy mid-career fellowship project Dementia Talking: Care, Conversation and Communication. She is the author of over 100 publications in critical social and health psychology, including *Psychologies of Ageing: Theory, Research and Practice* (Palgrave Macmillan, 2018, with Carol Holland and Michael Murray).

Damien W. Riggs is Professor in Psychology at Flinders University. He is the author of over 200 publications on gender, family and mental health, including (with Shoshana Rosenberg, Heather Fraser and Nik Taylor) *Queer Entanglements: Gender, Sexuality and Animal Companionship* (Cambridge University Press, 2021).

Louise Ritchie is Professor in Dementia Research and Director of the Alzheimer Scotland Centre for Policy and Practice at the University of the West of Scotland. She is a psychologist who is interested in interdisciplinary collaborations and involving the voice of people with lived experience. Her research focuses on understanding the experience of living with dementia and co-produced interventions to improve the lives of people living with dementia, their families and people who care for them. Her most impactful research projects relate to dementia and employment; improving the employment-related support available to people living with dementia post-diagnosis. A full list of projects and publications is available here: https://research-portal.uws.ac.uk/en/persons/louise-ritchie.

Melanie Rock's primary appointment at the University of Calgary is in the Department of Community Health Sciences. Since joining the University of Calgary two decades ago, she has drawn on her training in anthropology, health promotion and social work in research projects that combine human–animal studies with policy studies. The outcomes arising from Professor Rock's leadership include more than 100 scholarly publications, as well as policy influence in Canada and internationally.

Lorena Sordo is Postdoctoral Scholar at the University of California, Irvine. She obtained her PhD in 2021 from the University of Edinburgh, where she studied feline cognitive dysfunction syndrome (aka feline dementia), primarily focusing on age-related neuropathological changes and their similarities to Alzheimer's disease. During this time, she also investigated ways to diagnose feline dementia through imaging techniques, such as MRI, and potential interventions to reduce its clinical signs. Her current research interests include characterising age-related neuropathologic changes, identifying biomarkers that could aid in the diagnosis of early stages of neurodegenerative diseases, as well as recognising novel natural models for the translational study of Alzheimer's disease and other neurodegenerative diseases.

Nik Taylor conducts research on mechanisms of power and marginalisation expressed in/through human relations with other species informed by critical/intersectional feminism. Nik is currently Co-Director of the New Zealand Centre for Human-Animal Studies at the University of Canterbury, New Zealand, where she also teaches topics in the Human Services programme that focus on human–animal violence links; scholar-advocacy; social change, and crime and deviance, particularly domestic violence and animal abuse. Nik's latest books include *Queer Entanglements* (Cambridge University Press, 2021, with Damien Riggs, Heather Fraser and Shoshana Rosenberg) and *Rescuing Me, Rescuing You: Companion Animals and Domestic Violence* (Palgrave, 2019, with Heather Fraser).

Ann M. Toohey holds an Adjunct Assistant Professor appointment in the University of Calgary's Department of Community Health Sciences and also managed the University's Brenda Strafford Centre on Aging from 2017 to 2023. Her research programme explores the health promoting potential of human–animal relationships later in life and their ethical and public health implications for ageing-in-place. This interest has led her to explore the complexities of using animatronic pets with older adults living with dementia.

Stuart Woods is an immunologist, parasitologist and Lecturer in the School of Health and Life Sciences, University of the West of Scotland. His research is focused on the host pathogen interaction with a particular interest in

Toxoplasma gondii infection. Stuart's research has contributed to knowledge on host–pathogen interaction and in the development of a novel platform technology for the targeted delivery of therapies for infection. This work has generated 28 peer-reviewed publications which can be viewed here: https://research-portal.uws.ac.uk/en/persons/stuart-woods.

Preface and acknowledgements

This edited collection of essays, state-of-the-art reviews, research reports and provocations is the most significant output of the Multi-Species Dementia International Research Network so far (https://multispeciesdementia.org/). Established in October 2019, the network is the first of its kind to bring together researchers from across continents, disciplines and career stage to explore how we might build a more multi-species approach to understanding dementia. The network arose from an initial workshop that we organised in May 2019 on the theme of 'Multi-Species Dementia Care: Current Practice & Future Possibilities', which was held at the University of the West of Scotland's Lanarkshire campus, which overlooks the picturesque Campsie Fells. Fifty-eight people attended the workshop – a mixture of academics, health and social care practitioners, funders, policy makers, animal welfare representatives and people with lived experience of dementia. Clearly, we felt, there was interest in multi-species thinking and a desire across a broad spectrum of people to see how such thinking could help shape dementia care research, policy and practice.

It was not long after the establishment of the network, and only a matter of weeks before we were due to hold our first face-to-face meeting, that the global pandemic brought on by the emergence of SARS-Cov-2 brought major disruption to academic networking and collaboration. As countries across the world entered a series of national lockdowns, we were forced to move our network activities entirely online. This was not an easy process, as many of us were unfamiliar with videoconferencing technologies and with collaborative online platforms. Despite these challenges, we have managed to develop as a network and over the course of the pandemic have been able to develop our ideas and our contributions to this edited collection.

We are grateful to our funders who have been instrumental in supporting us at various stages of our development. We would like to thank the British Society of Gerontology for funding our initial workshop, and the Wellcome Trust for supporting the establishment of the network and our initial networking activities. We would also like to thank our current funders, the Royal Society of Edinburgh, for their generous support. We have been assisted by various human and more-than-human actors, including Maple the goat and Uno the dementia dog, who helped to make our initial workshop such a success. We are grateful to all who have helped to inspire this volume, especially those whose lives and (multi-species) relationships have been affected by dementia.

1

Introducing multi-species dementia studies

Nicholas Jenkins, Anna Jack-Waugh and Louise Ritchie

Dementia beyond the 'human'

On 27 April 2016, Lizzie Hill from Surrey, UK asked online readers of the *Guardian* newspaper, 'Do other mammals suffer from dementia and Alzheimer's disease?'[1] The 44 publishable responses to Lizzie's question ranged from the serious, to the personal, to the frankly ridiculous. *TSJones*, for example, posted that 'Dementia is a disease of the brain. Essentially it is a gradual death of brain cells – a neurodegenerative disorder – so any being which has a brain is likely to experience a dementia under certain conditions.' Others, like *Reframe*, replied, 'Silly question [*sic*] Haven't you ever had an old cat?' *Fatboyslimmer* commented that, 'My budgie is thick as f*ck these days', which prompted *Wisewinton* to ask, 'These days? So has he demonstrated dazzling intelligence before?'

Thinking about dementia across species lines, as Lizzie was doing, typically provokes such a mixture of interest, enthusiasm, scepticism, mockery and derision. All too often unconscious anthropocentrism[2] blinds us to the ways in which dementia connects, entangles and binds us with other living beings. As editors, we wanted to explore what ways of knowing dementia might be being closed off, when we come to rely upon anthropocentrism and the 'human' as our primary frame of reference. We wanted to know what a less anthropocentric and more multi-species approach to dementia might look like. This edited book is an attempt to explore this unfamiliar terrain.

Why, readers may very well ask, is anthropocentrism problematic when it comes to dementia? On the one hand, the answer to that question is fairly simple: because we do not live in a mono-species world. Across human societies and throughout human history, we humans have worked, lived, learned, played, aged and died alongside members of other species (Ritvo, 2007). It stands to reason then, that if dementia affects 'us' it will also have widespread and far-reaching implications for 'them'. In our search for cures and disease modifying forms of therapy, for example, we have created new, transgenic species of mice and fruit fly, whose very existence is rooted in our desire to eradicate dementia. Beyond the laboratory, we are increasingly enlisting the assistance of other animals, such as dogs and horses, in the care of people living with dementia. Many people with dementia share their homes, their lives and their dementia journeys with companion animals who, in the words of Boris Levinson (1972: 101), play 'an important role in the psychological economy of the retiree'. Members of other species, in other words, are already 'on the scene', yet we often fail to attend to them, and fail to see the significance of their presence, when we view dementia through a human-centric set of lenses. The second, and more complicated answer, is that what we consider to be 'human' (*anthropos*) is not fixed but changes across cultures, societies and over time; and that how we understand what it is to be human has fundamental implications for how we in turn seek to understand dementia. Prior to the European Enlightenment (1685–1815), for example, humans were positioned within the Great Chain of Being (see Lovejoy, 1964). Derived from the writings of Plato and Aristotle, the Great Chain viewed Being as hierarchical and multi-layered, reaching from the permanent and ethereal (the realm of God and angelic entities) to the temporal and material (the realm of humans, animals, plants and minerals). Within the Great Chain, beings were linked to those above and below them through the sharing of common attributes. Humans were thought to possess angelic qualities, such as the capacity for love and language, as well as bestial attributes in that humans have a material body that hungers, thirsts and lusts. Further, within the Great Chain, the boundaries between layers of Being were viewed as permeable, rather than impermeable. A human could thus elevate upwards towards the angels or descend downwards, towards the beasts. It was this belief system, following Scull (1979) and Foucault (1967/2001), that formed the lens through which dementia and other forms of 'insanity' were viewed during the pre-modern era. Insanity, within the logic of the Great Chain, signalled a descent into animality, and a corresponding fall from the status of Man. In contrast, the dawn of the European Enlightenment and the rise of liberal humanism led to a distinctly modern sense of the 'human' as a subject who is ontologically distinct, exceptional and set apart from the rest of existence (Foucault, 1970). It was through this new frame of reference that dementia became reconceptualised as an ailment of the human condition; one that could be studied scientifically, treated and, ultimately, cured (see, for example, Pinel, 1806). While this undoubtably led to progressive changes in how people affected by dementia are regarded, an important corollary of coming to see dementia through our liberal humanist frame of reference is that our very understandings of what dementia is have become inseparable from our (very modern) understandings of what it means to be 'human'.

In preparing this edited volume, we are not proposing a return to the Great Chain of Being or to a similar, pre-Enlightenment understanding of dementia. Rather, we are hoping to move *beyond* our reliance upon liberal humanism, and upon human exceptionalist ways of thinking, in order to develop ways of understanding dementia that are less wedded to the belief that human beings are set apart from all other species. In so doing, we may come to see that members of other species may well have something useful to teach us, not only about dementia, but about what it means to be human.

What we mean by multi-species

In May 2023, we searched ISI Web of Science[3] for all academic outputs across all disciplines and research fields that used the term *multi-species* (or *multispecies*) in the title, abstract or keywords. We were looking to see how the phrase had been used within academic publishing and across academic disciplines, since the term was first deployed in 1946.[4] Our search of the database returned a total of 15,636 entries.

It seems that some of the first scientific papers to use the term appeared during the early 1960s within the fields of chemical physics (Fromhold, 1963) and clinical pathology (Wisecup and Crouch, 1963). For the next two decades, the term appears to have been little used by researchers, with only 123 outputs recorded between the years 1963 to 1983. During the 1990s, however, use of the term appears to have increased sharply. By 1994, over 100 outputs using the phrase were being recorded annually within the ISI's database; a trend which appears to continue during the early 2000s. By 2018, however, over 1,000 outputs using the term were being recorded annually (see Figure 1.1).

Figure 1.1: Total number of outputs recorded each year with the term multi-species or multispecies in either the title, abstract or keywords, ISI Web of Science

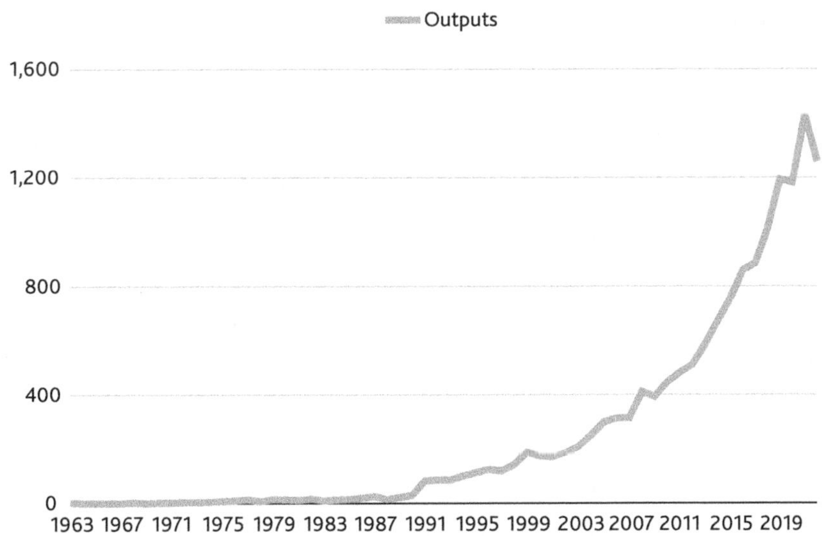

This seemingly dramatic increase in the use of the phrase among researchers may be explained, in part, by the proliferation in academic publishing that has taken place since the mid-20th century. As the total number of academic outputs being published across all areas increases, so arguably will the number of outputs that use a relatively specialised term. While this may be the case, our search suggests that the use of the phrase has not simply increased but has diversified within academic publishing, especially since the 2010s.

From the 1960s to the present, the phrase multispecies (or multi-species) appears to have been used predominantly by researchers working within the natural sciences. Of the total 15,636 outputs that we identified, 4,379 (28 per cent) were published in the fields of Ecology and Environmental Science alone. When the phrase is deployed within these fields, it appears to serve a largely pragmatic function, simply indicating the presence of two or more species of biological organism within the scope of inquiry. As the term enters the lexicon of the humanities and social sciences during the 2010s, however, it comes to adopt a distinct set of ethical, epistemological and methodological implications (see, for example, Kirksey and Helmreich, 2010). These implications, we have come to refer to as *multi-speciesism*.

Following van Dooren et al (2016), multi-speciesism involves more than merely incorporating two or more species of biological organism within the scope of inquiry. Rather, we believe multi-speciesism is best understood as an emergent philosophical worldview. In other words, as a way of approaching being, knowing, ethics and methodology that is distinct from that which is prescribed by the established worldviews of *(post)positivism*, *constructivism*, and *pragmatism* (Creswell and Creswell, 2018). In contrast to these human-centric worldviews, multi-speciesism is guided by an emphasis on decentring the human as the main focal point of inquiry and in situating human beings, human societies, human cultures and human problems within a much broader set of worldly relations. These relations invariably involve a multiplicity of beings continuously learning how to 'get along' with each other on a planet that is becoming both fragile and precarious (Haraway, 2008; 2016).

We believe that there are (at least) three principles that serve to distinguish multi-speciesism as a distinct philosophical worldview: entangled reciprocity; multi-species worldings; and, response-ability. Entangled reciprocity refers to the assumption that all living beings are connected to other living beings in ways that are not simply transactional, but generative. In other words, from a multi-species perspective, relations between members of one species and another are made possible, not because each has something to gain from the other, but through the mutual histories and shared heritages that knot together species in complex processes of co-becoming (Haraway, 2008). By attending to these mutual histories and shared heritages, we gain insights into multi-species worlds as complex webs of lively exchange that are perpetually changing, and within which different forms of life are continuously *becoming-with* each other (Haraway, 2008; 2016). Processes of entangled reciprocity form the basis of multi-species worlding. This assumes that our worlds are neither objectively real nor subjectively ideational. Rather, they are the product of a 'material-semiotic interplay' (van Dooren et al, 2016: 12) in which ways of knowing are not passive but agential and part-and-parcel of the world's becoming (Barad, 2007). In other words, the ways in which members of different species come to 'know' their worlds has material consequences, as their knowledge affects the very composition of the worlds they inhabit. Thus, knowing and being, ontology and epistemology, are, from a multi-species perspective, inseparable. Because of this, multi-species researchers are not tasked with simply understanding multi-species worlds. Multi-species inquiry is neither interpretive nor objective, but perpetually entangled within and acting upon the multi-species worlds that the researcher inhabits and is seeking to know. The stories we tell about our worlds *matter*, in both a semiotic and a material sense, because our stories form part of our response-ability (Haraway, 2016). Response-ability, we believe, is a key concept within multi-species inquiry. It refers not to the ethical obligation to act, but to the capacity to respond, with others, in the creation of multi-species worlds that we are *for*. This is because, as van Dooren et al (2016: 16) argue, '[a]t the end of the day, decisions must be made about how we will get on inside a world that is, however multiple, also shared, finite, and (in many ways) struggling'.

This brief and inevitably somewhat cursory overview of multi-species thinking brings us to a fundamental question: What do *we* mean by multi-species in the context of dementia? At its most basic level, we believe it means thinking about dementia as something that affects *more* than humans alone. It means attending to the ways in which scientific understandings of conditions like Alzheimer's disease are predicated upon our relations with other species, and asking ourselves what new forms of knowledge and what new ways of knowing might become possible, should those relations develop in new and hitherto unexplored directions. It means becoming curious about how age-related neurocognitive disease may be experienced by other mammals, aside from humans, and to ask ourselves how these experiences may call upon us to respond. It means exploring how human experiences of dementia may be shaped by multi-species relations that take place *under* the skin, within the human body, and to ask ourselves how knowledge of such relations may be useful, not only in preventing and ameliorating neurocognitive conditions, but in reconfiguring our understandings of embodied subjectivity itself; as a complex landscape within which relations between the human and more-than-human are continuously taking place. It means expanding our understanding of 'family' or 'kin' for people living with dementia and to explore the ways in which relations between humans and other sentient beings form part of the broader, multi-species, psycho-social sequelae of neurocognitive disease. And it means exploring how changes in incidence, prevalence and mortality in dementia may be shaped by broader, systems-level changes in planetary conditions, especially those caused by anthropogenic processes such as global warming and fossil fuel consumption. It means, in short, refocusing the *lens* of the dementia debate (Bartlett and O'Connor, 2007; 2010) in ways that seek to bring our relations with other living beings and the wider planet into much sharper relief.

The future contours of multi-species dementia studies

At the height of the COVID-19 pandemic, we published our first article on multi-species dementia studies (Jenkins et al, 2021). The article was developed as an online collaborative project, involving members of the Multi-Species Dementia International Research Network.[5] Through collaborative writing, we were seeking to chart the key contour lines of what may become a distinctly multi-species approach within contemporary dementia studies. We have had time to refine our thinking since the publication of that article and, in the subsections that follow, we offer a summary of four key terrains within which multi-species approaches have potential to produce new insights, new contributions and lead to new ways of doing things (differently) in dementia.

Dementia pathology and illness experience

Biomedical understandings of what dementia is and how dementia develops are shaped by, and mediated through, multi-species relations. As Davies, Gorman and Milne highlight in Chapter 2, since the 1990s our attempts to understand the pathogenesis of Alzheimer's disease have been based largely on research involving non-human subjects, especially transgenic mice. The knowledge acquired through these animal 'models' has, over the years, been presented as both scientific breakthroughs and as sources of frustration and disappointment. Rarely, however, do we investigate the processes through which such knowledge is generated. There are some understandable reasons for this. As Tamagnini et al (2018) highlight, those working within the laboratory may be wary of talking openly about their use of animals in biomedical research, while social scientists have largely avoided engaging with the aetiology of neurocognitive disease, choosing instead to focus on the dementia disease experience. Critical engagement with how scientific knowledge about dementia is produced through multi-species relations, and translated for human benefit, is vital. The efficacy and ethics, for example, of breeding animals and insects for dementia research are complex, yet little is known about how scientists navigate these thorny terrains or about how those affected by dementia feel about the use of animal bodies 'in their name'. Outside of the laboratory, many non-human mammals display signs of neurocognitive disorder as they age. Indeed, the existence of Cognitive Dysfunction Syndrome (CDS) in other species has been acknowledged within veterinary science since the 1990s (for example, Landsberg and Ruehl, 1997; Borras et al, 1999). According to Prpar Mihevc and Majdič (2019) the similarities in pathology between Alzheimer's disease in humans and CDS in other mammals are such that these could well be two facets of the same disease. Despite this, dementia studies has largely ignored age-related neurocognitive disorder when it is present in non-humans. Why has this aspect of dementia been so systematically neglected within our field? Following Arluke and Sanders (1996), we suspect the failure to attend to dementia across species is due more to a reliance upon anthropocentric thinking than on robust data or empirical analysis. Such thinking tends to assume that as only humans can experience and become affected by dementia, there is nothing useful to be gained by attending to neurocognitive disorder in other species. As Sordo highlights in Chapter 3, this is clearly not the case and much may be gained by attending to how age-related neurocognitive conditions, that we call dementia, manifest themselves across the more-than-human world. However, while there are many benefits to be gained, cultivating multi-species understandings of dementia pathology and illness experience will, of course, not be easy. Researchers must tread a careful line. They must avoid anthropomorphising animals while, at the same time, not zoomorphising the experiences of people living with dementia. Following Despret (2013), we believe that attending to difference, broadening our methodologies while always acknowledging the perpetually partial nature of our understandings will be central considerations.

Care and caring

Multi-species work has the potential to reshape our understandings of what care is and of how caring is accomplished in the presence of dementia. Care is a notoriously 'slippery' concept (Martin et al, 2015). While it is talked about extensively in relation to dementia, it is surprisingly difficult to pin down with any degree of precision or uniformity. In policy and practice communities, care is typically defined in pragmatic terms; as, for example, 'activities and relations involved in meeting the physical, psychological and emotional needs of adults and children, old and young, frail and able-bodied' (International Labour Organization, 2018: 6). Within feminist scholarship, by contrast, care takes on much broader significance. According to Fisher and Tronto (1990: 40), for example, it is 'a species activity that includes everything we do to maintain, contain, and repair our "world" so that we can live in it as well as possible'.

Whether it is understood as the accomplishment of practical tasks or as a way of *Being-in-the-world*, when discussed within dementia studies care has tended to be conceptualised as an interpersonal (human-to-human) mode of relating. This stems largely from the field's reliance upon humanistic psychology. From a humanistic perspective (for example, Rogers, 1967/2004), what defines certain practices as care is not the behaviours themselves, but the meanings that such behaviours are intended to convey. In other words, through the performance of certain behaviours, there is interpersonal recognition of a unique and exceptional *Self* that is being cared for, and held in regard, by an equally unique and exceptional *Other*. As Jenkins, Jack-Waugh and Ritchie highlight in Chapter 7, this is not the only form of care that is on display within dementia settings, yet multi-species caring is often ignored, or anthropomorphised within 'person-centred' and 'relationship-centred' approaches to dementia. In contrast, multi-species approaches tend not to conceptualise care as the outcome of interpersonal recognition, but rather, as the capacity for empathetic connection that includes yet extends beyond human beings. Notions of 'entangled empathy' (Gruen, 2015) and 'embodied empathy' (Despret, 2013), for example, understand care as rooted in the body's capacity for empathetic awareness which goes beyond putting oneself 'in the shoes' of someone else; especially, as Gruen (2015: 61) highlights, 'animals do not wear shoes!' Empathetic practice is a mode of attending that involves inquiring into the embodied position of the Other – of what the world looks like, sounds like, smells like and feels like from *this* embodied position – and, from there, asking ourselves how we may be being called upon to respond. As Jenkins, Jack-Waugh and Ritchie highlight in Chapter 7, this way of thinking can provide important insights when exploring experiences of 'animal assisted' forms of dementia care, especially in conditions where interpersonal recognition is not part of the therapeutic equation. And yet, while important, consideration of care as an empathetic mode of attending goes beyond the study of animal assisted interventions. It requires deliberate and careful cultivation of a body's desire to know (more) about the embodied positions of animal *Others*, who have largely been ignored within mainstream dementia studies. In Chapters 5 and 6, for example, Peel, Riggs and Taylor and Ashall, respectively, care about the experiences of aged canine family members living with CDS. Through their care, they explore the ways in which ageing and neurocognitive decline is experienced within animal bodies and the various ways in which their experiences call upon us, as humans, to respond.

Dementia, self and environment

Multi-species thinking offers an approach to exploring connections involving dementia, our selves and our environments, in ways that are qualitatively distinct to those that have tended to dominate dementia studies since the 1980s. As Peel, Riggs and Taylor highlight in Chapter 5, and Jenkins, Jack-Waugh and Ritchie highlight in Chapter 7, before the 1980s it was not uncommon for dementia to be likened to 'a funeral that never ends' (Aronson and Lipkowitz, 1981: 569). The Personhood movement of the 1980s and 1990s was one of the first to challenge this orthodoxy. It asserted that 'loss' of self was due more to 'the unconscious defenses, compulsions and interpersonal processes that pervade this field of work' (Kitwood, 1997: 5) than to neuropathology. From a Personhood perspective, loss of self in dementia represents a failure of interpersonal recognition. In other words, a failure of care. While this way of thinking has brought increased attention to care environments, it has been underpinned by the liberal humanist ideal of the self, as a uniquely human form of subjectivity that is set apart from others and from the natural world. As the social anthropologist Clifford Geertz notes, this is 'a rather peculiar idea within the context of the world's cultures' (Geertz, 1975: 48).

Multi-species perspectives have the potential to recast our understandings of the self and of the relations between selves, environments and dementia. As Crilly, Woods and Henriquez highlight in Chapter 4, our bodies are rich environments of multi-species relations and scientific research is increasingly coming to understand how relations within, for example, the microbiome affect the onset and progression of dementia disease. As Jenkins, Jack-Waugh and Ritchie argue in Chapter 7, these new scientific understandings lean towards a view of the self that has been recognised within non-Western civilisations for centuries. Within this view, selves are understood as porous (as opposed to impermeable), relational (as opposed to autonomous) and transactive (as opposed to static) (Marriot, 1976; Strathern, 1988; Nhat Hanh, 2017). As such, self and other, human and non-human, internal and external are not seen as binary opposites but as entangled; the other exists within the self, the non-human exists within the human, the external exists within the internal. In Jenkins et al (2021) we argued that the emergence of the pathogen SARS-Cov-2 and the global COVID-19 pandemic that followed highlighted a pressing need to recast our approach to the relationship between dementia, selves and environments. In the UK alone, estimates suggest more than one in five deaths linked to COVID-19 (21.8 per cent) were among people living with dementia (Office for National Statistics, 2022). As de Wit et al (2020) argue, the emergence of new pathogens like SARS-Cov-2 may be a direct consequence of broader changes to the planetary environment, such as global warming, declining biodiversity and declining natural habitats, which are themselves the direct consequences of anthropogenic activities, in particular modern farming, deforestation and fossil fuel consumption. Ageing and physiology alone do not explain the increased vulnerability that people with dementia experienced during the pandemic. Decisions to discharge people with dementia from hospitals to care homes without testing for COVID-19 (Willet et al, 2020) and to restrict access to ventilators based on perceived 'frailty' (National Institute for Health and Care Excellence, 2020), among others, contributed directly to excess deaths. Thus, by exploring how pathogenic viruses emerge from anthropogenic processes and become entangled within immune systems, amyloid plaques, ageism and cognitive ableism, we reach beyond the humanistic emphasis on interpersonal recognition, and the immediate care environment, and towards a 'whole-systems' perspective.

Rights, power and personhood

Multi-species approaches have the potential to create new modes of political activism in dementia. According to Bartlett (2012), the early 2000s witnessed the *emergent* modes of dementia activism. These modes, Bartlett argues, were characterised by the creation of campaigning organisations run by and for people with dementia, such as the Scottish Dementia Working Group, the Dementia Engagement and Empowerment Project (DEEP) and Dementia Alliance International. Underpinned by a social model of disability and a Human Rights Based Approach, these emergent modes have campaigned for dementia to be recognised as a disability like any other, and for people living with dementia to access their rights as enshrined within national and international charters (see, for example, Hughes and Williamson, 2019; Shakespeare et al, 2019).

Prior to the emergent modes of dementia activism, those concerned with the ethical treatment of animals have also drawn upon the language of rights as a framework for political mobilisation. The animal liberationist Peter Singer (1975/2015), for example, argues that our willingness to extend rights to marginalised populations while, at the same time, withholding them from other sentient beings speaks to the prevailing influence of speciesism across Western societies. In an attempt to align speciesism with other forms of discrimination, including ableism, calls have been made to extend those rights typically afforded to human 'persons' to members of other species who, like humans, possess the capacity to experience suffering (Singer, 1975/2015) or who may be considered the subject of a life (Regan, 1987).

Despite both drawing upon rights-based frameworks, dementia activism and animal activism have developed as separate spheres of concern. In recent years, however, researchers, scholars and activists have started to highlight points of connection between ableism and speciesism, as interlocking forms of oppression, and to argue that much could be gained from synthesising these spheres of political activism. Santinele Martino and Lindsay, for example, argue that:

> Disabled people bring rich perspectives around inter-dependence, creative ways of mobilising, and making space for non-normative ways of voicing lived experience. At the same time, critical animal studies can contribute to disability studies scholarship and activism through its extensive work on advocating for the 'voiceless' through a holistic approach, which considers all beings and environments, through our social relationships and unavoidably interdependent existences. (Santinele Martino and Lindsay, 2020: 2–3)

In this context, multi-species thinking offers a rich terrain within which to explore new affinities and potential alliances. What it may offer both spheres of activism is an opportunity to move *beyond* the language of citizenship and rights, as these continue to rely upon anthropocentric notions of exceptionalism. In so doing, it may enable us to explore how personhood and power in dementia are made within the mundane processes of entangled reciprocity and of multi-species world-making. This way of thinking, however, is something of a radical departure from the now established, as opposed to emergent, modes of dementia activism. As such, some within the movement may be understandably wary of losing hard-won ground in the fight for rights and for inclusion of dementia within social models of disability. What multi-species thinking offers in this respect, is not a replacement of one form of activism with another form of activism, but an alternative for those who see connections between speciesism and ableism and who want to see new worlds in which all species flourish.

The structure of this book

The chapters contained within this edited book speak directly to the contours of a multi-species dementia studies, as outlined in the previous section, although not necessarily in discrete, sequential or discipline-specific order. Our first three chapters explore the role of multi-species relations in shaping scientific understandings of dementia. The first of these chapters, by Davies, Gorman and Milne, considers the role of transgenic mice in the 'fabrication' of scientific understandings of Alzheimer's disease. Their use of the term fabrication is not meant to imply scientific knowledge of dementia is made up, although they do highlight attempts by certain scientists to fraudulently claim results from animal models. Rather, drawing on scholarship within Science and Technology Studies, Davies, Gorman and Milne use fabrication as a theoretical lens through which they explore how everyday decision-making, taking place continuously within scientific communities, comes to position certain theories of Alzheimer's disease causation, and their corresponding routes to treatment, as more plausible and as preferable over others. From this stance, Davies, Gorman and Milne argue that the fabrication of the amyloid cascade hypothesis, which is now the dominant theory of Alzheimer's disease causation, has been predicated upon a series of decisions, through which patients with rarer forms of Alzheimer's disease first come to stand in for those with more common forms of the disease and, second, where transgenic mice come to stand in for humans. Maintaining this fragile alignment between the brains of mice and the brains of people, Davies, Gorman and Milne argue, has very real consequences for the future of scientific research. However, in an era where funders request, expect and require people affected by dementia be involved in reviewing scientific proposals and in decision-making, Davies, Gorman and Milne also point to new and emergent possibilities. Patient representatives, they argue, are becoming more aware of the reliance upon mouse models in dementia science and becoming adept at reading, with caution, the promises of translation and of new therapies that mouse models are thought to offer. Patient representatives, they argue, appear keen to open up dementia research to new possibilities, beyond amyloid cascade hypothesis based mouse models, so as to embrace a wider variety of hypotheses, methodologies and needs of patients living with dementia.

The next chapter builds on the possibilities of knowing dementia beyond mouse models. In Chapter 3, Sordo highlights that transgenic mice are far from being the only models available to scientists to understand dementia pathogenesis. While the genetic make-up of laboratory mice must be altered for them to develop dementia neuropathology many other species produce such changes spontaneously as they age. In a manner accessible to the non-specialist, Sordo describes systematically how neuropathological processes that have long been observed in the brains of humans living with Alzheimer's may be observed (albeit with important differences) in the brains of dogs, cats, leopards, cheetahs, donkeys, dolphins and wolverines, among many others. In addition to comparable processes in neuropathology, Sordo also highlights the ways in which mammals, aside from humans, display changes in cognition and behaviour that appear to result from neuropathogenesis, and which can be observed clinically and measured using standardised instruments. This leads Sordo to an important conclusion, which is that 'it is impossible to look into AD without referring to cognitive decline and/or dementia in animals, and vice versa'. Attending to dementia's 'interspecies similarities', Sordo argues, has mammalian implications, as it may 'facilitate interventions that can improve the quality of life of human and animal elder populations'.

Building on the theme of imagining new scientific possibilities, in Chapter 4 Crilly, Woods and Henriquez take the reader 'under the skin' to explore how immune systems and central nervous system relate with microbiomes and pathobiomes in dementia. Traditionally, Crilly, Woods and Henriquez highlight, the central nervous system was considered an 'immunologically privileged site', in which the blood brain barrier prevents microorganisms – such as bacteria, viruses and protozoa – from taking up residence or exerting influence. This view, they argue, is challenged by a developing hypothesis that sees infection and inflammation as playing key roles in the development of neurological conditions, including Alzheimer's, Parkinson's and frontal-temporal dementia. What emerges through their discussion is an understanding of human immunity as a complex and changing relationship involving human host and symbiotic microbial communities. Commensal microbes, they argue, are an intrinsic part of humans' 'front line defenses' against infection. Yet, when harmony is disrupted by the presence of pathogenic microbes – such as *Toxoplasma gondii, Helicobacter pylori* or influenza – the immune system triggers a variety of pro-inflammatory, anti-inflammatory and regulatory responses; ostensibly through the production of a group of proteins called cytokines. These, Crilly, Woods and Henriquez highlight, have been shown to affect neurons on both a short-term and longer-term basis. Further, they argue, these intra-corporeal processes become entangled with the ageing process through *inflammaging*; a concept first proposed by immunologist Claudio Franceschi to describe how cytokine production elevates as humans age. We humans, Crilly, Woods and Henriquez argue, become more 'inflammatory' the older we get. Inflammaging, they highlight, is a complex interplay involving genetics, environments, microbes and immunological processes. As such, relations between infection, inflammaging and dementia are likely to be highly complex and are, so far, only partially understood. What is needed, they argue, is a much more holistic approach in which nervous systems are seen as complex landscapes within which relations between microbes, neurons, ageing and dementia are taking place.

The next two chapters turn from biomedical understandings, towards issues of care, caring and the multi-species psycho-social sequelae of dementia. In so doing, they each explore how love and loss in dementia are experienced within the context of multi-species family life. Also referred to as more-than-human families (Irvine and Cilia, 2017) multi-species families are familial networks within which non-human beings are 'incorporated into the family within a caring, parental relationship or as pack members' (Solhjoo et al, 2022: 1093). Drawing upon their own experiences of living within multi-species families, in Chapter 5, Peel, Riggs and Taylor explore the nature of love and loss when caring for canine family members experiencing CDS. These are family members who, the authors readily acknowledge, 'others might not recognize as worthy of love and/or might undervalue the love we have for them'. Informed by critical kinship studies and critical posthumanism, Peel, Riggs and Taylor apply a 'queer menagerie' approach to examine what is displayed when each of them writes about dementia as experienced by family members they have loved and lost. What emerges through their reflexive writing challenges pronatalist understandings of family and kinship, in which childbearing and human–human relations tend to be centred. In so doing, it offers insights into how personhood, love, time, death and loss in dementia may be experienced within a 'queer family formation'. What, Peel, Riggs and Taylor ask, might we learn from decentring dementia as an exclusively human experience? One implication, they argue, may be a greater role for veterinarians, both in naming and claiming canine dementia and in supporting humans within multi-species families to enable their canine loved ones to live well with dementia.

Written within the post-qualitative tradition (St Pierre, 2019) and from the first-person perspective of a carer, scholar, activist and veterinary surgeon, in Chapter 6 Ashall explores multi-species experiences of loss, grief, and guilt during the COVID-19 pandemic. Here, Ashall seeks to diffract (Barad, 2007) her experiences of caring for and caring about canine and human family members as a 'provocation for us to think differently, beyond species boundaries, about what caring for those living with dementia could mean'. Starting with the painful realisation that Ashall's aged canine family member would have lived longer, had they survived into the first UK-wide lockdown during the summer of 2020, Ashall poignantly describes the feelings of guilt and grief that accompany decision-making in relation to canine euthanasia. From there, Ashall explores her experiences of how, during the same summer, a close family member with dementia was admitted to a care home, where they spent the last few weeks of their life. Through these moving and deeply personal accounts, Ashall describes how the death of a canine family member provided an affective landscape, and source of insight, which facilitated positive caring during the COVID-19 pandemic. 'What would it mean', Ashall asks, 'if we acknowledged, embraced or even positively encouraged cross species learning of the type that I have described?' For Ashall, as with Peel, Riggs and Taylor, there are clear implications for veterinary practice, especially in the extension of palliative care to non-human family members. Yet, following Puig de la Bellacasa (2017), Ashall also argues that recognition of our interspecies entanglements in dementia has implications that reach beyond practical end-of-life considerations and provides a deep source of speculative reimagining of what it means to care.

Building on the theme of reimagining care, the final two contributions explore the application of multi-species thinking within dementia theory and practice. In Chapter 7, Jenkins, Jack-Waugh and Ritchie explore how multi-species thinking may reinvigorate debates regarding personhood in dementia and inform the development of person-centred approaches to practice. Starting from an understanding of persons as multi-species holobionts, as opposed to autonomous 'individuals', Jenkins, Jack-Waugh and Ritchie explore how understandings of the body as a landscape of multi-species relations can lead to new forms of ethical appreciation and valuing that reach beyond the confines of liberal humanism. Turning next to the 'zoological dimension' (Bryant, 1979), Jenkins, Jack-Waugh and Ritchie consider human–animal interactions in dementia as rich sites of multi-species intercorporeality. Drawing on the reflexive accounts of Anne Rankin, a carer and activist who now lives with a Dementia Dog (Uno), they argue for an approach to doing person-centredness in dementia that is rooted in an ethic of response-ability. To practice response-ability, they argue, is to recognise the ways in which 'becoming in dementia is a world-making process in which entanglements of humans and animals are knotted and re-knotted in complex ways' and that by 'becoming with each other within shared conditions of response-ability, people affected by dementia and animals have the potential to form new relations which, in turn, give rise to new possibilities for becoming'. Following Haraway (2008), Jenkins, Waugh and Ritchie argue that personhood, mindedness and animality are 'at stake' when people with dementia and animal *Others* encounter each other within the everyday worlds of dementia and a successful outcome is far from guaranteed.

Resisting an entirely biocentric focus, Toohey et al explore the presence of animatronic robotic animals in dementia care, as the final contribution to this volume. Rapid advancements in the sophistication and affordability of robotic technologies, Toohey et al argue, are leading to animatronic companions such as those made by Joy for All™ becoming increasingly common within dementia care settings. Drawing on ethnographic fieldwork conducted in Canada during the COVID-19 pandemic, Toohey et al argue that feelings of ambivalence and discomfort were commonplace among family members of people with dementia, who engaged with robotic animals, especially when their loved ones had formed close affective bonds with these technologies. Such feelings, Toohey et al argue, were not as visible among staff working in dementia care facilities, who appeared used to seeing residents forming close attachments to inanimate objects, such as teddy bears or dolls. While this was the case, managing risk, reality and illusion were constant considerations within these human–robotic assemblages. In this context, Toohey et al argue that the introduction of 'animal-like' companions is troubling dementia care, because it disrupts humanist assumptions regarding, for example, what is 'real' and what is 'fake', what is 'human' and what is not, what is 'organic' and what is 'inorganic'. Because of this, and when viewed within humanistic frameworks, witnessing caring for robotic entities that do not require care may appear futile, infantilising or un-dignifying for the person with dementia. When viewed from a posthumanist perspective, however, Toohey et al argue that it makes visible a form of 'vibrant relationality' from which spontaneous acts of caring and the experiencing of affective companionship may emerge. Thus, if we suspend our reliance upon humanistic principles, Toohey et al argue, we may come to see that 'the ontological division between dignity and indignity in caring with, caring for, and caring about a robotic companion animal may be a false one'.

The need for interdisciplinarity

As may already be apparent through the summaries provided in the previous section, the contributions to this edited volume span a variety of disciplines, interests, concerns and specialist knowledge. In many ways, we see this as a strength and as a testament to the diversity and potential that multi-species dementia studies has to offer the wider field. Developing multi-species ways of thinking, researching and practising in dementia is a complex endeavour and one that sits outside the remit of any single academic discipline or specialism. Exploring the complex and multi-faceted ways in which dementia knots together the human and the more-than-human will require that we draw upon knowledge, concepts, methodologies and approaches from across the natural sciences, the social sciences, the arts and the (post)humanities. In many respects, the contributions contained within this volume offer a *multi*-disciplinary contribution to multi-species dementia studies, rather than an interdisciplinary one. Each contribution draws largely from its respective field and, when viewed as a single collection, there are clear differences in their approaches to dementia. We, as editors, have not sought to impose an artificial uniformity on these contributions or to create a false sense of intellectual coherence across them. Bringing our different perspectives and priorities together is a necessary first step, but it is by no means the end of the road. What is required, we believe, is a move towards a more interdisciplinary approach. While often viewed by academics, researchers, funders, policy makers and others as a *sine qua non* for innovation, interdisciplinarity is not an uncontested concept and not without its challenges and its critics. Scientists and artists must learn to speak each other's languages, and the points where epistemology, methodology and ethics meet can give rise to intense debates and to intense emotions. Arguably, the field of dementia studies is well suited to this challenge, given the variety of disciplines and bodies of knowledge that already contribute to it. While this is the case, some considerable movement may be required if we are to fully explore what a more multi-species understanding of dementia may have to offer. Those working within the social sciences, for example, may need to expand their often-limited understandings of 'the medical model' of dementia, in order to appreciate the diversity and multiplicity of knowledges that travel under that banner. Scientists equally, may need to expand their understandings of what constitutes 'data' or 'rigour' when understanding how artists and social scientists make sense of dementia's multi-species worldings. What we need as a community, and following Haraway (2008: 36), is to cultivate our own response-ability, in which we are prepared to become subject to an 'unsettling obligation of curiosity, which requires knowing more at the end of the day than at the beginning'. In the Afterword to this volume, we provide some practical suggestions and examples of how we might cultivate such response-ability, as we move towards a more interdisciplinary approach to developing multi-species dementia studies.

This book is not intended to be read in a linear format and readers may well wish to direct their attentions towards those chapters that speak to their interests and specialisms. We very much hope, however, that readers will feel tempted to engage with chapters that sit outside of their own disciplines, areas of expertise and comfort zones, and, in so doing, become 'curious' about what an interdisciplinary, multi-species dementia studies might have to offer.

Notes

1 'Is dementia unique to humans?' *The Guardian*, 27 April 2016. Available from: https://www.theguardian.com/lifeandstyle/2016/apr/27/is-dementia-unique-to-humans

2 Derived from the Greek word for human (*anthropos*), anthropocentrism refers to the tendency, especially within Western societies, to view humans as the central and most important beings in existence.

3 www.webofscience.com

4 According to Merriam-Webster online dictionary, https://www.merriam-webster.com/dictionary/multispecies#:~:text=%3A%20composed%20of%2C%20containing%2C%20or,a%20multispecies%20flock%20of%20birds

5 https://multispeciesdementia.org/

References

Arluke, A. and Sanders, C. (1996) *Regarding Animals*, Philadelphia, PA: Temple University Press.

Aronson, M.K. and Lipkowitz, R. (1981) 'Senile dementia, Alzheimer's type: The family and the health care delivery system', *Journal of the American Geriatrics Society*, 29(12): 568–571.

Barad, K. (2007) *Meeting the Universe Halfway: Quantum Physics and the Entanglement of Matter and Meaning*, Durham, NC: Duke University Press.

Bartlett, R. (2012) 'The emergent modes of dementia activism', *Ageing & Society*, 34(4): 623–644.

Bartlett, R. and O'Connor, D. (2007) 'From personhood to citizenship: Broadening the lens for dementia practice and research', *Journal of Aging Studies*, 21(2): 107–118.

Bartlett, R. and O'Connor, D. (2010) *Broadening the Dementia Debate: Towards Social Citizenship*, Bristol: Policy Press.

Borras, D., Ferrer, I. and Pumarola, M. (1999) 'Age-related changes in the brain of the dog', *Veterinary Pathology*, 36(3): 202–211.

Bryant, C. (1979) 'The zoological connection: Animal-related human behavior', *Social Forces*, 58(2): 399–421.

Creswell, J.W. and Creswell, J.D. (2018) *Research Design: Qualitative, Quantitative and Mixed Methods Approaches*, Thousand Oaks, CA: SAGE.

Despret, V. (2013) 'Responding bodies and partial affinities in human-animal worlds', *Theory, Culture & Society*, 30(7–8): 51–76.

de Wit, W., Freschi, A. and Trench, E. (2020) *COVID-19: Urgent Call to Protect People and Nature*, Woking: World Wildlife Fund.

Fisher, B. and Tronto, J. (1990) 'Towards a feminist theory of caring', in E.K. Abel and M.K. Nelson (eds) *Circles of Care: Work and Identity in Women's Lives*, New York, NY: SUNY Press, pp 35–62.

Foucault, M. (1967/2001) *Madness and Civilization: A History of Insanity in the Age of Reason*, London: Routledge.

Foucault, M. (1970) *The Order of Things*, London: Tavistock.

Fromhold, A.T. (1963) 'Space charge in growing oxide films. III. Multispecies diffusion', *Journal of Chemical Physics*, 39(9): 2278–2282.

Geertz, C. (1975) 'On the nature of anthropological understanding', *American Scientist*, 63(1): 47–53.

Gruen, L. (2015) *Entangled Empathy: An Alternative Ethic for Our Relations with Animals*, New York, NY: Lantern Books.

Haraway, D. (2008) *When Species Meet*, Minneapolis, MN: University of Minnesota Press.

Haraway, D. (2016) *Staying with the Trouble: Making Kin in the Chthulucene*, Durham, NC: Duke University Press.

Hughes, R. and Williamson, T. (2019) *The Dementia Manifesto: Putting Values-Based Practice to Work*, Cambridge: Cambridge University Press.

International Labour Organization (2018) *Care Work and Care Jobs: For the Future of Decent Work*, Geneva: ILO.

Irvine, L. and Cilia, L. (2017) 'More-than-human families: Pets, people, and practices in multispecies households', *Sociology Compass*, 11: e12455.

Jenkins, N., Gorman, R., Douglas, C., Ashall, V., Ritchie, L. and Jack-Waugh, A. (2021) 'Multi-species dementia studies: Contours, contributions and controversies', *Journal of Aging Studies*, 59: 100975.

Kirksey, S.E. and Helmreich, S. (2010) 'The emergence of multispecies ethnography', *Cultural Anthropology*, 25(4): 545–576.

Kitwood, T. (1997) *Dementia Reconsidered: The Person Comes First*, Buckingham: Open University Press.

Landsberg, G. and Ruehl, W. (1997) 'Geriatric behavioral problems', *Veterinary Clinics of North America Small Animal Practice*, 27(6): 1537–1559.

Levinson, B. (1972) *Pets & Human Development*, Springfield, IL: Charles C Thomas.

Lovejoy, A.O. (1964) *The Great Chain of Being: A Study of the History of an Idea*, Cambridge, MA: Harvard University Press.

Marriot, K. (1976) 'Hindu transactions: Diversity without dualisms', in B. Kapferer (ed) *Transaction and Meaning: Directions in the Anthropology of Exchange and Symbolic Behavior*, Philadelphia, PA: Institute for the Study of Human Issues, pp 109–142.

Martin, A., Myers, N. and Viseu, A. (2015) 'The politics of care in technoscience', *Social Studies of Science*, 45(5): 625–641.

National Institute for Health and Care Excellence (2020) 'COVID-19 Rapid guideline: Critical care in adults', *NICE*, 20 March. Available from: https://www.nice.org.uk/guidance/ng159 [Accessed 11 November 2020].

Nhat Hanh, T. (2017) *The Art of Living: Peace and Freedom in the Here and Now*, New York, NY: HarperCollins.

Office for National Statistics (2022) 'Deaths due to COVID-19, registered in England and Wales: 2021', *ONS*, 1 July. Available from: https://www.ons.gov.uk/peoplepopulationandcommunity/birthsdeathsandmarriages/deaths/articles/deathsregisteredduetocovid19/2021 [Accessed 27 June 2023].

Pinel, P. (1806) *A Treatise on Insanity*, London: Messrs, Cadell and Davies.

Prpar Mihevc, S. and Majdič, G. (2019) 'Canine cognitive dysfunction and Alzheimer's disease – two facets of the same disease?', *Frontiers in Neuroscience*, 12(13): 604.

Puig de la Bellacasa, M. (2017) *Matters of Care: Speculative Ethics in More Than Human Worlds*, Minneapolis, MN: University of Minnesota Press.

Regan, T. (1987) 'The case for animal rights', in M. Fox (ed) *Advances in Animal Welfare Science 1986/87*, Boston, MA: Martinus Nijhoff Publishers, pp 179–189.

Ritvo, H. (2007) 'On the animal turn', *Daedalus*, 136(4): 118–122.

Rogers, C. (1967/2004) *On Becoming a Person: A Therapist's View of Psychotherapy*, London: Constable & Robinson Ltd.

Santinele Martino, A. and Lindsay, S.M. (2020) 'Introduction: The intersections of critical disability studies and critical animal studies', *Canadian Journal of Disability Studies*, 9(2): 1–9.

Scull, A. (1979) 'Moral treatment reconsidered: Some sociological comments on an episode in the history of British psychiatry', *Psychological Medicine*, 9(3): 421–428.

Shakespeare, T., Zeilig, H. and Mittler, P. (2019) 'Rights in mind: Thinking differently about dementia and disability', *Dementia*, 18(3): 1075–1088.

Singer, P. (1975/2015) *Animal Liberation: A New Ethics for Our Treatment of Animals*, London: Bodley Head.

Solhjoo, N., Krtalić, M. and Goulding, A. (2022) 'Pets and people: Information experience of multispecies families', *Journal of Documentation*, 78(5): 1092–1108.

St Pierre, E. (2019) 'Post qualitative inquiry, the refusal of method, and the risk of the new', *Qualitative Inquiry*, 27(1): 3–9.

Strathern, M. (1988) *The Gender of the Gift: Problems with Women and Problems with Society in Melanesia*, Berkeley, CA: University of California Press.

Tamagnini, F., Cotton, M., Goodall, O., Harrison, G., Jeynes, C., Palombo, F., et al (2018) 'Of mice and dementia: A filmed conversation on the use of animals in dementia research', *Dementia*, 17(8): 1055–1063.

van Dooren, T., Kirksey, E. and Münster, U. (2016) 'Multispecies studies: Cultivating arts of attentiveness', *Environmental Humanities*, 8(1): 1–23.

Willet, K., Winn, M., Roughton, R. and Skinner, A. (2020) 'COVID-19 hospital discharge service requirements', *NHS England*, 19 March. Available from: https://www.england.nhs.uk/coronavirus/publication/covid-19-hospital-discharge-service-requirements/ [Accessed 11 November 2020].

Wisecup, W.G. and Crouch, B.G. (1963) 'Evaluation and calibration of an electronic particle counter for enumeration of multispecies blood cells', *American Journal of Clinical Pathology*, 39(4): 349–354.

2

Fabricating mice and dementia: opening up relations in multi-species research

Gail Davies, Richard Gorman and Richard Milne

Introduction

This chapter was written during a moment of flux in the unravelling of the plaques, tangles and tales that characterise over 30 years of research for treatments of dementia involving humans and animals. In the autumn of 2022, there were widely circulated reports in the mainstream media of a pharmaceutical breakthrough following long periods of investment in the so-called 'amyloid cascade hypothesis' (ACH). This focused on the small benefits in slowing cognitive decline for some people using the drug lecanemab. While modest, the results were reported as a significant success: ending 'decades of failure' and promising a step towards 'a new era of drugs to treat Alzheimer's' (*BBC News*, 2022). However, even amid celebrations there were cautions about the wider potential of this drug, which could only be given to people with early Alzheimer's disease who had evidence of amyloid plaques from scans or spinal fluid analysis, excluding the 98 per cent of people who were untested, many other types of dementia and those in the later stages of disease (Walsh et al, 2022). The success of lecanemab had been constructed, or fabricated, through careful articulation of the relations between one version of dementia, the associated animal models, targeted drug pathways and a particular patient population. Yet, this highly specific 'scientific breakthrough' (Brown, 2000) achieved extensive celebratory media currency after many years of unfulfilled expectations for all those hoping for a cure for dementia.

We use the story of this scientific breakthrough to frame our exploration of the organisation of translational research on dementia using mouse models of Alzheimer's disease. We are interested in how the trajectories of drug development tightly knit together particular animals, humans and drug pathways by focusing on the specific biological processes that can be modelled, evidenced and altered in multi-species experimental systems (Davies, 2010, 2013b; Milne, 2020). We are also interested in the forms of dementia and other ways of doing research that fall outside of these biological pathways. While the therapeutic breakthroughs enabled by the ACH are to be celebrated, they raise a challenging issue for constructing multi-species dementia in biomedical research. Bringing animal models in the laboratory and humans in the clinic into sufficiently close relations so that manipulations in one organism effectively model processes relevant to therapeutic outcomes in another means bracketing off alternative research options and the multiplicity of human experiences of dementia. Making decisions about which animal model to progress has implications for both the animals used in research and the humans affected by this health condition. We are interested in how we might tell stories about research and drug development that are more accountable to the multiplicity of people and animals' lives they touch.

We use the concept of how mouse models are 'fabricated' in dementia research to focus attention on these processes of decision-making in science. We use this concept to unpack how disease models are fabricated as a way of bringing the decisions made by researchers in specific research trajectories into conversation with the decisions made by people affected by dementia who are reviewing new research proposals for medical charities. We explain our use of the concept of fabrication more fully in what follows, but note here that we consider fabrication an important process in all scientific research in which decisions to focus on certain things give shape to the tools, techniques, animals and evidence that are built into research pathways. Yet we use the term acknowledging it can have a pejorative meaning too. These processes are fallible and open to other kinds of fabrication and forgery that reflect motivations and methods in science; though malfeasance is only a small part of the uncertainties around reproducible and responsible science (Macleod and the University of Edinburgh Research Strategy Group, 2022). The stories of dementia research contain irresponsible behaviour as well as successful breakthroughs for science; repeatedly deferred hope as well as expectations realised for people affected by dementia.

We start by discussing our use of the concept of fabrication and introduce the research we draw on in this chapter. We then present two different ways of telling stories about the organisation of multi-species biomedical research on dementia. First, we trace the experimental practices used to construct mouse models within the ACH. This focuses on how researchers fabricate the animals and patient populations that link and make visible the specific biological pathways they hope will make a difference to disease trajectories. Second, we explore how people affected by dementia, acting as patient representatives in reviewing proposals for new biomedical research, locate themselves and their families within these stories of recurrent hope and delayed promise. We explore how they relate to the animals they encounter in research proposals and their responsibilities to others affected by dementia. While the future biomedical research trajectories of the ACH are underpinned by the translations made possible by transgenic animals based on specific family genomes, the patient representatives we spoke to wanted to acknowledge a wider set of relations, drawing attention to the importance of equity and balance to benefit those affected by Alzheimer's disease now. We conclude by reflecting on the different dimensions of accountability in dementia research and the challenge of working between multi-species relations and the multiple versions of dementia.

Fabricating animal models in biomedical research

Animal models have played a pivotal role in the development of research on dementia in humans to date (Götz and Ittner, 2008). Currently much of this research takes place using fruit flies (drosophila) and specially bred strains of genetically altered mice (Vitek et al, 2020). These animal models do not attempt to recapitulate the whole human experience of disease but to develop an experimental model of a specific aspect of the condition that researchers hypothesise is of relevance to the way that the disorder emerges and develops in human brain tissue. Fruit flies are often used to research the genetic factors that may underpin certain forms of dementia; linking breeding experiments that alter genes and the spatial behaviour of these small insects. Mice have been used to explore the potential links between altered brain tissue and cognitive function; including through the protein plaques in the ACH introduced earlier. Working with flies and mice mean that many generations of animals can be bred in laboratories and many aspects of biology altered in ways that would be impossible with research in humans. Yet every animal model is limited in the aspect of the disease that it isolates. Every animal model is thus a speculative hypothesis about how altering a specific aspect of the condition may have implications for the production of a disease altering treatment. We can thus say that all animal models are fabricated or manufactured to work within the specific experimental system in which they are located.

In talking about how animal models are fabricated in dementia research, we are building on two bodies of work in Science and Technology Studies (STS). First, we draw on a now extensive literature by social scientists and philosophers tracing how animal models of disease are constructed in different places and for different purposes (Ankeny and Leonelli, 2018). These case studies focus on the manufacture of different animals historically, as in the development of mice models for early cancer research (Rader, 2004) or models using rats to research alcoholism (Ankeny et al, 2014), to the production and use of mice in more recent research in psychiatry and neuroscience (Davies, 2010; Nelson, 2018), functional genomics (Davies, 2013a) or immunology (Davies, 2012). These studies demonstrate how models are highly situated experimental interventions that involve manipulating the capacities of animals and coordinating action across different communities of research, connecting the places where models are developed and assured (Davies, 2013b; Parry, 2020), the databases collating information on animals for research communities (Leonelli and Ankeny, 2012), to the cross-species exchange that enables insights generated in one animal (here mice) to move to another (humans) for new clinical treatments (Leonelli, 2012).

The use of any animal model thus involves a series of research decisions (Dietrich et al, 2020). These include which animal model to use for the next stages of research; how many animals to use in an experiment; when to move from the animal model to work in humans; or when to move from one animal model to another when research trajectories change. In focusing on decisions, we want to connect to a second body of work in STS on selectivity in the making of knowledge. While researchers do face decisions around which model, including animal models, they might use in their next experiment, the historical processes through which certain animal models of dementia have become woven into research trajectories may not always be evident at the moment of planning new experiments. Each earlier decision shapes the scope for future choices. As STS scholar Knorr-Cetina suggests, 'the products of science are not only decision-impregnated, they are also decision-impregnating, in the sense that they point to new problems and predispose their solutions' (Knorr-Cetina, 1981: 229). Knorr-Cetina uses the term fabrication explicitly in her work on how decisions taken in the laboratory create opportunities for certain scientific 'facts' to travel outside of the laboratory, foreclosing other ways of understanding an issue.

Fabrication has at least two meanings in everyday language: how things are manufactured through putting things together in new ways, or how things are fraudulent or faked. As we explore in this chapter, both processes can be identified in the longer histories of research using mouse models in dementia, as in many other scientific fields. Both draw attention to the methodological choices made by researchers as they forge new research projects. Both are also consequential for the outcomes from this research. In our first story we demonstrate how the scientific trajectories and outputs in dementia research may have been shaped by questionable data from animal models, but we are most interested in how processes of everyday fabrication in science construct pathways around certain animal models, as these feature in successful research proposals, are most frequently published in the academic literature, best characterised in the database, or used to provide evidence for subsequent clinical trials. These choices become deeply entangled in the complex experimental systems of science (Rheinberger, 1997) and are stabilised in the distributed 'decision-making networks' through which biological researchers, funders, journals and national governments shape the direction and design of biomedical research processes (Caron-Flinterman et al, 2007). Knorr-Cetina suggests that as 'scientific facts are fabricated in the sense that they are derived from decisions, they can be defabricated by imposing alternative decisions' (1981: 6). However, making decisions about things like animal models in laboratory research is usually considered the domain of experts, and it is not clear how or where alternative questions could be asked, or alternative decisions imposed in 'upstream science' when the social consequences of technological choices are hard to predict (Marris and Rose, 2010).

In what follows we are also interested in how looking at processes of fabrication could be used to open up the potential for patient and public involvement (PPI) to shape decisions in health and care research, including around dementia (Gove et al, 2018). Researchers are now expected to involve the people affected by their work in key decisions throughout the 'pipeline' of their research, from building partnerships with patient groups, to determining research priorities, or organising clinical trials (Wilson et al, 2015; Maccarthy et al, 2019). Yet, there are still many questions around how patient participation might affect decisions within biomedical research, in part due to what Caron-Flinterman et al call the 'resilience of the biomedical decision-making network' (2007: 339) outlined earlier. There is now more advice on how to involve patients and others affected by health conditions in biomedical research (Shared Learning Group on Involvement, 2016; Davies et al, 2022). However, there are still enduring challenges. These emerge from the uncertain value of patient participation for institutions, the specialisation of biomedical research communities and the often still marginal position of patient groups in relation to the wider socio-technical networks of biomedical research (Caron-Flinterman et al, 2007). In our second story, we suggest that they also emerge from the way that certain animal models have become embedded in research trajectories 'black boxing' or truncating the apparent options for making alternative decisions. These animals shape research trajectories; yet their material forms mean they are seen as less amenable to the deliberative methods that undergird patient participation and there are assumptions about how far their role in research can be questioned and who has the capacity to open up these issues (Davies et al, 2024a).

We can give further shape to the process of following fabrication in science by borrowing from work in related fields. In their study of the fabrication of government accrual accounting systems, Bruno and Lapsley (2018; see also Preston et al, 1992) draw on foundational work by Latour and Woolgar (1979) to open up the often opaque material processes through which private sector business practices become adopted in public services, including health. They explore how experimental forms of accounting become implemented through distinct stages of fabrication. In outline they summarise:

> The notion of fabrication is articulated in three 'images,' and includes three different concepts. These are as follows: to build (the process of construction); the fragility (the weakness that could result in a failure); machinations (which tell convincing stories about the system and indicates the plan to sell the new system benefits and purpose to skeptics). (Bruno and Lapsley, 2018: 1051)

They use the term fabrication not to suggest that such methods are necessarily flawed or indeed fraudulent, but to indicate how their implementation requires complex and continual processes, including storytelling. They focus on the processes of building models, recognising their fragility, and improvising the narratives that secure their value. Fabrication, they write, is chosen rather than construction, as it includes both the essential fragility of methods of construction and the machinations required to make them work (Bruno and Lapsley, 2018: 1052). We suggest the processes of fabrication summarised here may be usefully applied to the complex histories of constructing animal models in dementia research. The threefold schema of fabrication can be used to open up discussions about how animal models are constructed in biomedical research, how their limitations are acknowledged and managed, as well as the narratives that are circulated about them in the scientific press and elsewhere. Such stories tightly link together research practices and patient communities, shaping the multi-species relations and 'regimes of hope' that give shape to the fabrication of research trajectories (Moreira and Palladino, 2005; Moreira, 2009).

In what follows we bring two social science research projects together to explore the tales told about animal models of dementia and consider ways of opening up fabrication processes to those with a stake in these stories. First, we expand on the development of the ACH in research on Alzheimer's disease. We explore how this animal model was constructed, identify moments of improvisation, and consider how it has endured through stories of success, failure and even fraud to place a particular multi-species relation at the centre of much research on dementia. Milne's past work has explored the emergence, development and 'calibration' of animal models over the last 40 years of Alzheimer's research (Milne, 2020). His research draws attention to how mouse models have acted as the basis for translating research conducted with families with rare genetic forms of Alzheimer's disease into the development of novel therapeutics for common, sporadic forms of the condition. We then look at how a wide range of patient representatives understand their role in reviewing applications for new biomedical research on dementia. Davies and Gorman's work has explored the growth of PPI in laboratory animal research (Davies et al, 2020; Gorman and Davies, 2020), including looking at how patient representatives review research proposals that use animal models. Bringing these projects together enables us to explore how multi-species relations are made in dementia research, and how people affected by dementia are placed in several ways through these processes, only some of which they are aware of and thus able to affect.

Aligning humans and animals in Alzheimer's research

The fabrication of animal models of Alzheimer's disease involves building models and narrating connections, continually shoring up fragile research relations. We are particularly interested here in the alignments this has generated between different forms of dementia and different mammalian species. The first enables patients with rare forms of Alzheimer's disease to stand in for those with common forms. The second enables mouse models that recapitulate the molecular pathologies associated with the ACH to act as sufficiently good avatars, or models, of disease. The challenge of aligning both establishes a fundamental tension in biomedical research between how to characterise the multiple versions of dementia and how to move, or translate, between multiple species.

When Alzheimer's disease was first described in 1907, it was as a presenile form of dementia characterised by neuropathological evidence, including the presence of 'plaques', 'tangles' and the loss of neurons. Alois Alzheimer, and subsequently Emil Kraepelin, emphasised the onset of Alzheimer's disease in comparatively young people, distinguishing it from senile dementia. However, by the 1960s, it was possible to argue, following pathologist Woodard, that: 'Most pathologists dealing directly with this problem tend to consider the two entities [Alzheimer's disease and senile dementia] as basically identical' (Woodard, 1966: 1157). Historian Ballenger similarly argued that, while Alzheimer's disease was 'officially' a rare form of pre senile dementia, 'every researcher of this period seriously engaged in the study of dementia was aware that Alzheimer's disease and senile dementia were for all practical purposes the same entity' (Ballenger, 2006: 118).

This practical alignment was formalised through a combination of new techniques, clinical reclassification and the emergence of a social movement that engaged political interest in diseases of ageing. In the process, narratives of Alzheimer's disease transitioned from those of a rare disease worthy of case reports in neurology or psychiatry journals to a leading cause of death (Fox, 1989; Beard, 2004; Ballenger, 2006). Key to this shift was a 1977 meeting between four US bodies responsible for research funding, including the US National Institute for Ageing (NIA) and the National Institutes of Health (NIH). NIA director Robert Katzman later explained how this acted both 'to reach consensus that Alzheimer's disease (AD) was not just a relatively rare neurodegenerative disorder of the presenium, but was the major cause of dementia in the elderly in developed countries' and to 'bring together investigators … to help "jump-start" research in AD' (Katzman and Bick, 2000: xi).

This reclassification of clinical disease in humans was accompanied by the reconstruction of biomedical research in animals. By the end of the 1980s, Alzheimer's disease had settled on a 'theory-methods' package, which combined the techniques of molecular biology and human genetics with the molecularised theory of disease causation known as the ACH, introduced earlier. Elaboration of the ACH model of disease established molecular links between the pathologies found in the brains of patients with both familial (or genetic) and sporadic forms of Alzheimer's disease. The ACH was set out in its classic form by Hardy and Higgins (1992) in a review describing a potential biological mechanism for the changes associated with Alzheimer's disease, combining Hardy's work on families with genetic forms of disease and Higgins' evidence from experiments using transgenic mice. Higgins and colleagues purported to have created mice whose brains produced disease relevant amyloid precursor proteins, and to have shown that this single change could lead to the neuropathology – the plaques and tangles – distinctive to Alzheimer's disease.

This mouse model apparently demonstrated that mice could mimic the biological changes seen in people with the familiar forms of Alzheimer's disease who were the focus of work by Hardy and colleagues. These 'transgenic amyloid mice', demonstrating what John Hardy called 'fulminant Alzheimer pathology, both plaques and tangles' (2006: 152), became a key 'tool' in furthering research around ACH from the late 1980s. Alignment between humans and animals was achieved through foregrounding this particular aspect of biology, side-lining other biological, social or environmental influences on human and animal experience (see also Davies, 2010). Higgins' mice appeared to support this emphasis, locating Alzheimer's disease in the biology of mouse and human brains, while constructing equivalence between both species of disease (familial and sporadic) and species themselves (here humans and mice).

However, the fabrication of animal models achieved by Higgins and colleagues was not, it emerged, limited to the construction of relationships, but also involved invention. The *Nature* paper describing the mouse model was later retracted. In his 2006 retrospective, Hardy suggested his co-author on an influential paper setting out the ACH, Gerry Higgins, had not only contributed to constructing transgenic mice, but also faking the evidence of the expression of disease relevant proteins in mice. As Hardy recounts: 'As the probable fraud of [Gerry's] mouse analysis was uncovered, he resigned, left science and disappeared. So this paper, while it could be seen as the beginning of the amyloid cascade hypothesis, was Gerry's last' (Hardy, 2006: 152). Yet, the research trajectory based on the ACH continued even as the probable forgery around the mouse model was made public.

It was not until 1995 that a 'robust' mouse model of Alzheimer's disease pathology was developed, in the form of the PDAPP, or APP^{V717F} transgenic mouse, reported by the Californian biotech company Athena Neurosciences (Duff, 1999). These mice reproduced a specific genetic variant in the amyloid precursor protein identified in a family in Indiana and came to form the basis for drug development throughout the 1990s and early 2000s (Milne, 2020). However, the strength of the analogic relationship between human and mouse brains, and between familial and sporadic forms of disease, continued to be contested, not least as drugs developed using these models failed to show effects. Fabricating a successful model for research on Alzheimer's disease necessarily involved construction, fragility and narration; but there were few success stories to report. As one participant in a 2012 NIH forum put it, although 'we can cure amyloidosis in transgenic mice with hundreds of compounds', there are no 'animal models of a neurological or psychiatric disease that are faithful to the disease itself' (Greenberg, 2012: 58).

The lack of successful treatments developed on the basis of the ACH represented a significant challenge to the successful fabrication of the associated mouse models, highlighting their fragility in moving data and drugs meaningfully between patient and animal bodies. Improvising around the model again, the criteria for patient inclusion of clinical trials began to change to improve alignment. Throughout the recent history of Alzheimer's disease research most studies, including clinical trials, were conducted with 'people with dementia', identified in clinics as being at different stages of clinically symptomatic illness (Moreira, 2009; Milne, 2018). However, constructing a better alignment between disease and potential drugs in the research pathways opened up by the ACH has involved enrolling newly specified kinds of patients, based on realigned relations of biological equivalence. Specifically, the failure of drug trials has been integral to the redefinition of diagnostic criteria for Alzheimer's disease over the last decade, establishing measures such as abnormal levels of beta-amyloid and tau proteins as biological markers of disease that *precede* cognitive and behavioural symptoms (Milne and Latimer, 2020). This process enrols people understood as being 'at risk' or even as having 'preclinical' Alzheimer's disease into the research process, building new relations between animals and new kinds of patients, as well as prompting new kinds of narratives that emphasise prevention and anticipation (Hampel et al, 2022).

This realignment is evident in the recent approvals by the US Food and Drugs Administration of the first potential 'disease-modifying' drugs for Alzheimer's disease: aducanumab (or *Aduhelm*) and lecanemab (or *Leqembi*). Both these drugs reduce levels of amyloid and aim to prevent the development or progression of symptoms. Their approval reinforces research trajectories built around the specific biological characteristics shared between human and mouse models established through the ACH.

The initiation of clinical trials for aducanumab and lecanemab were based on evidence from the *Tg2576* and *Tg-ArcSwe* mouse models (Mullan et al, 1992; Nilsberth et al, 2001), which overexpress mutant forms of the amyloid precursor protein due to specific mutations associated with rare early onset forms of the disease found in single extended families. Both lecanemab and aducanumab focus on patients with 'early' stages of symptomatic disease, namely mild cognitive impairment and mild dementia, even as the clinical status of the former – and its value as a diagnostic label for patients – remains unclear (Beard and Neary, 2013; Saunders et al, 2022). They also require patients to have biological evidence of this form of the disease, in the form of abnormal levels of beta-amyloid protein. It is this that allows the fragile relationship between common, late-onset forms of Alzheimer's disease and the rarer, early-onset forms, to persist.

Moving this biological equivalence to the centre of decision-making has involved (in the United States at least) a reworking of Katzman's consensus to place the ACH at the heart of the disease experience. Despite its fraught history of construction, fragility and even fraud, recent stories of success help fabricate a more wide-reaching animal model. In the United States, the Alzheimer Association, a leading organisation representing patients and caregivers, has enthusiastically embraced and sponsored revisions to the diagnostic criteria for this disease. It has actively mobilised in support of the newly approved drugs through launching the 'More Time' campaign to attempt to influence the Food and Drugs Administration's decision, coordinating the inclusion of patient and caregiver testimony within the advisory review (Joseph, 2021). The newly emerging coalition of advocacy organisations, pharmaceutical companies and academic researchers that has formed around aducanumab and lecanemab strengthens the fabrication process described earlier – bolstering the fragile links built around rare forms of disease and narrating them into the future of healthcare. Telling a story of success through the ACH requires narrowing down the ways that people, animals and drug pathways are brought together in dementia research. While there is multiplicity in dementia itself and many ways in which it can be studied in health and care research, the current focus of research using animal models in the ACH reduces this complexity. In this context, multi-species dementia turns out to look rather singular.

Opening up to patient perspectives on dementia

We now turn to a separate set of perspectives on the construction, fragility and narration of animal models in Alzheimer's research, drawing on qualitative interviews with people affected by dementia in the UK. While the earlier section looked at the highly specific relations drawn between certain humans and animals through the biomedical research trajectories around the ACH, here we examine how people affected by dementia seek to engage with different forms of multiplicity when making decisions about new biomedical research. We draw on our work within the Animal Research Nexus Programme, which looked at the changing interfaces between patient involvement and animal research, and involved talking to people affected by dementia who had volunteered to review new biomedical research proposals for medical research charities (Gorman and Davies, 2020; Davies et al, 2022; Davies et al, 2024b). Patient involvement with laboratory research is still a relatively new node in the 'biomedical decision-making network' (Caron-Flinterman et al, 2007) we introduced earlier. There are many questions about how and how far it might contribute to the way scientific trajectories might be 'defabricated' (Knorr-Cetina, 1981), or refabricated, in response to the perspectives of people in whose name research is carried out.

In our work, we surveyed researchers and those involved in reviewing biomedical research and conducted in-depth interviews with 22 patient representatives, 20 scientists, and 17 involvement and engagement professionals. We also organised events bringing these different stakeholder perspectives together. The people we spoke to who were reviewing research proposals drew on experiences as carers or patients with many kinds of dementia including vascular dementia, frontotemporal dementia (FTD), as well as Alzheimer's. Many had been involved in reviewing research for many years. Rather than adopting the singular identity or position of a 'person affected by dementia', many also drew on professional backgrounds in the health services, the civil service, consultancy, business and third sector management to evaluate biomedical research. When reviewing research planning to use animal models to study dementia, they asked a range of questions about the organisation of research trajectories. Many felt they had become adept at reading the stories of translational promise told by scientists around a single project and wanted to contextualise these narratives in multiple different ways. They sought to challenge researchers to learn in new ways from the failure of animal models, multiply research pathways, incorporate the range of experiences of dementia and rethink collaborative measures of scientific success. We present some of these perspectives here, using the pseudonyms allocated to participants and organisations in the Animal Research Nexus Programme (see Davies et al, 2024b).

These challenges were accompanied by a general acceptance of animal research, respect for scientists' skills and recognition of the constraints of contemporary science. The people affected by dementia we spoke to were volunteering time and expertise to support successful biomedical research. Many saw themselves as responsible allies and important members of a wider scientific effort but were also willing to question accepted ways of doing things. They sought to learn, understand and locate themselves and their families within scientific stories of hope and promise. They were interested in assisting scientists to construct effective models for dementia research, but they brought different things into their assessment of model fragility. They were often critical of the stories told in research proposals that presented the singular importance of any study as the next step. We introduce some criteria used to evaluate these proposals in what follows, including translatability from the patient perspective, equity in accessing the outcomes of research, and balancing investments across cure and care for people with dementia now.

Many people affected by dementia we spoke to were comfortable talking about how animal models were built into research trajectories and used in translational research. Over time they felt they had gained meaningful knowledge of how researchers used multiple mouse models in research. Through repetition they also acquired understanding of the fragility of these models and the continual need to improvise and improve the way they worked. As Toby explains:

> I have myself learned along the way quite a lot. And one of the areas is ... understanding what mouse models are, how researchers use them. That knowledge I've developed as a result of being involved in the network. ... Until I got involved in the [organisation], I didn't appreciate how many different types of mouse models there are. ... You increasingly realise there are limitations with all the different types of models. But of course, those discussions and that work needs to happen to improve the models themselves. (Toby, interview, 2018)

While they were not in a position to raise more technical questions around the fabrication of transgenic amyloid mouse models, many people questioned how researchers were responding to the continual failure of the ACH to generate clinical treatments at the time of interview. They questioned how effective it was to focus repeatedly on this specific hypothesis and its associated animal models. This was not a straightforward rejection by most, but a desire to open up questions about the allocation of resources and reduce waste – including in the use of animals – when resulting drugs continued to show results in mice but not humans. As Tabitha exclaims:

> I'm really struggling at the moment because everything they do in mice is not translating to humans. So, there's two things there. One is, is the [organisation] just throwing good money after bad every time it funds work using mice as the vehicle? [Second] That's a load of mice being killed totally unnecessarily because they're learning stuff, but it doesn't help find a cure for Alzheimer's. I've yet to be convinced. What I think they should be researching is why does it work so well in a mouse and not translate into humans, instead of carrying on doing all the basic research they're doing into tau and amyloid and all that

> sort of stuff because OK, they're finding all these drugs that you know. I want to come back as a mouse! Then I know if I get Alzheimer's as a mouse, they're going to cure me! But why throw money at it till you understand whether or not you really are learning anything from using mice? (Tabitha, interview, 2018)

Tabitha asks questions about translatability in ways that puts the patient rather than the hypothesis or animal model first. She exclaims she wants to come back as a mouse to benefit from existing research on Alzheimer's. She asks for work on translation exploring why the mouse model fails for many, rather than how to make it succeed for a few, focusing her disappointment on the ACH. For a few, this frustration spilled over into rejection of all proposed research in this trajectory: 'there's a lot with Alzheimer's about amyloid hypothesis, well I never believed in that hypothesis' (Tracy, interview, 2018).

Concerns about the translatability of research based on mouse models associated with the ACH led to people affected by dementia trying to open up alternative pathways around research. Tracy explains her frustration in having reviewed repeated proposals, with similar experimental models, premised around a singular vision of what treating dementia might look like. She describes her sense that funding bids 'felt narrow in what they were looking at because they had this bizarre idea of *a* cure' (Tracy, interview, 2018; original emphasis). Tina puts her critique of the singular vision that emerges from this version of multi-species dementia research in a similar way: 'When I look at the studies that come through for funding, there's just a huge amount looking at finding *the* cure, finding *the* treatment and it seems to be there's a bit of a mismatch there' (Tina, interview, 2018; original emphasis).

Many people who questioned the ACH mouse models wanted to see a wider diversity of biomedical research, including studies in humans, tissue cultures or using stem cell research, which they felt were underrepresented in the work they reviewed.

> When I look at the amount of funding that goes into using animal models, if that money was pushing to trying to recruit more humans, both in terms of maybe longitudinal studies, lifestyle, long-term lifestyle studies or maybe looking at tissue biopsy or scanning studies. … I tend to question quite avidly, why would a mouse model be useful in this particular situation? Why can't the researchers be looking for an alternative model, maybe a stem cell? (Tina, interview, 2018)

The promise of a singular research pathway did not accommodate their experience of repeatedly reviewing proposals that made grand promises about a cure, or the multiple dimensions of dementia that were important to them. People's responses were motivated by a complex mix of expectations for new research on the condition that affected them, but also for connection to multiple others, reflecting the responsibility and accountability to wider communities that comes through being affected by illness (Cartwright, 1998). For example, Rachel describes her initial focus in looking through proposals for research that reflected her personal experience of dementia: 'I saw some research that was very strongly linked to FTD, and it looked pretty ground-breaking, looking at the very specific proteins and a proposal that to me offered hope for the particular condition my husband had' (Rachel, interview, 2018). Yet, she later goes on to explain her growing feelings around the importance of 'trying not to just do a job where you're representing people with FTD but where you've got some awareness of all the dementias' (Rachel, interview, 2018). Many people we spoke to understand their contribution to involvement as extending from personal experience to wider patient advocacy incorporating equity of access to the outcomes of research into their evaluation. This sense of responsibility to others affected by different dementias was understood as a challenge for researchers: 'you've got PPA [primary progressive aphasia], PCA [posterior cortical atrophy], FTD, you can go on and on, there are so many different dementias now' (Tanya, interview, 2018). Yet they were concerned not to find this multiplicity reflected in the research they reviewed.

Others responded to stories of recurrent hope and delayed promise through biomedical research by seeking to rebalance organisational efforts from *a* future cure to a diversity of ways of helping people affected by dementia now. They referred to the importance of improving life with dementia and for the carers of those with dementia, and better resourcing of health and care research, alongside new biomedical studies. As Win describes:

> Because of our involvement as carers, we encouraged research, and the research programme, to be on the care side, not only medication based, or 100% the science and pathology of dementia. So over 10 or 15 years, we helped to balance it, to about 30% each of care, cure, and medicine, so these are all spread out. (Win, interview, 2018)

When reflecting on how they sought to balance all of the different responsibilities that they felt when reviewing proposals – towards the people affected by dementia in their lives, towards others with dementia and at times towards animals too – many people began to challenge how researchers were weighing these priorities in their decisions. The contribution they wanted to make extended from adding their lived experience to existing research trajectories to wanting to engage in dialogue about the underpinning assumptions organising research. Rachel suggests that scientists were falling short. She recognises her dependence on biomedical trajectories, but questioned how research pathways were organised to protect careers rather than improve care: 'There are real people who really need some solutions and that kind of protecting things so that you can make a name within the science world, at the expense of collaborating and getting to the end game quicker, there is something in that that could make me quite angry' (Rachel, interview, 2018). Others echoed this through an emphasis on the silo structures in biomedical research: 'I think sometimes people can be stuck in their own little world of research, once you've decided you're going into a certain area of work, then sometimes it's quite difficult to step outside' (Tina, interview, 2018).

Win's story shows how people affected by dementia do have the ability to alter the direction of dementia research, through rebalancing the allocation of organisational resources. Yet, opening up the trajectories of biomedical research is more challenging. There are several assumptions about the role that people affected by health conditions might play in reviewing laboratory animal research that make this more difficult (Davies et al, 2024a). However, we also found some scientific researchers welcoming the critical scrutiny of patient groups and their role in opening up how research decisions were made and how they might measure success.

> I've been encouraged by the fact that the patient groups are getting engaged and getting more savvy and recognising the difference between just getting another publication, which could be a lot easier than getting a publication that has some translational relevance to a particular disease area. … That's the fundamental thing that needs to change, is how we measure success. It's what is the output you're measuring and maybe we need to measure collaborations. (Ian, scientific researcher, interview, 2020)

Our work revealed the multiple forms of accountability that people affected by dementia saw as important in shaping research trajectories in ways that were shared by some researchers. As dementia researchers are increasingly expected to involve the people affected by their work in decision-making processes (Pickett and Murray, 2018), these conversations are likely to proliferate. This will require attention to how responsibilities and accountabilities are distributed at the intersection between spaces of patient involvement and animal research (Gorman and Davies, 2020). Opening up to patient perspectives on dementia has the potential to bring new opportunities and challenges for aligning animals in Alzheimer's research, but also requires multidisciplinary research able to articulate the multiplicity of dementia with multi-species dementia.

Conclusion

Both animal research and research on dementia are complex and contested fields, in which tensions are always near the surface. We have used recent stories of scientific breakthrough to open up the 'black box' of animal models of dementia and reflect on how these tensions are embodied in the processes of fabricating models through the construction, fragility and narration of research practices. First, we explored how relations between different species were brought together through the trajectories built around the ACH. Here, we focused on the multi-species practices of dementia research as it moves from laboratory animal models, through clinical trials, into potential human patients, providing an individual and evidential link between this animal model and this version of dementia. Second, we traced the way in which people affected by dementia evaluate scientific proposals, seeking to open up to the multiplicity of ways of experiencing and understanding dementia. Translational research on dementia has to work both across multiple species (here mainly mice and humans) and the multiplicity of this disease (including Alzheimer's, but also vascular dementia, and many others). We suggest many tensions in this field emerge from the difficulty of holding these different dimensions together and being accountable to the different agencies – animals, researchers and patients – with a stake in how this is done. Looking at how animal models are fabricated through processes of construction, improvisation and narration helps reveal how research trajectories are forged through the decisions made and stories told about research pathways, opening up questions around motivations and the way that accountability is imagined and enacted by different groups.

In closing we want to reflect on what a more accountable version of the fabrication of multi-species dementia research might look like for our research participants. The people affected by dementia we spoke to did not seek to take animals out of the pursuit of better outcomes from dementia, but they did want more open, authentic and ongoing dialogue about how animals were used in research (for a practical guide see Davies et al, 2022). They recognised the construction and fragility of these models, but wanted to have more open conversations about how they were narrated. Research involvement tends to position people affected by dementia as 'end-users' of a single research project, but many felt responsibilities for the multiple patient communities and the multi-species commonalities that are both included and excluded in particular research trajectories. They valued the opportunity to support research and play a more active role in decision-making processes, but this needs to be genuine. Too often 'patients' are asked to comment or give their assent to research when the story about what it means to fabricate a successful animal model in that area has already been closed down.

Many researchers we spoke to accept these challenges privately and were beginning to consider them more publicly. Acknowledging the fragility of fabrication processes can help researchers reflect on the histories and assumptions embodied in the animal models they use, the relationship between those animals and human forms of dementia, and the likelihood that this will impact on translation. What emerges from bringing these two social science projects together is the value of bringing together researchers and people affected by dementia to learn more about the histories and cultures of dementia research. People affected by dementia would prefer to know that a researcher wants to use a particular animal model because of their expertise, rather than be told that such a mouse is *the* only model to use; or that the current trajectory of biomedical research is the only option for their experience of dementia. Our interviews pre-date the recent stories of breakthrough around ACH, but many patient representatives have been here before. Both researchers and people affected by dementia recognise that animal models are constructed, and understand their fragilities, but their stakes in the stories told about them and their responses differ. The challenges raised by those taking part in PPI, and reading the promissory narratives of translational research, recapitulate the narrowing of trajectories built around the ACH through the focus on specific types of dementia and species of research. Both researchers and people affected by dementia are starting to ask questions about the wider benefits of multidisciplinary collaboration. Bringing these perspectives together could open up opportunities to tell more accountable stories of how animal models are positioned in relation to the multiplicities of dementia and the wider contexts of multi-species research.

Acknowledgements

We would like to thank Nick Jenkins and Anna Jack-Waugh for their invitation to contribute to this volume and their helpful comments on an earlier version of this chapter. Gail Davies and Richard Gorman would like to thank the patient representatives, involvement professionals and research scientists who contributed to their work, and acknowledge support of colleagues on the Animal Research Nexus Programme. Their research was supported by the Wellcome Trust [205393/Z/16/Z]. Richard Milne's work was also supported by the Wellcome Trust [220540/Z/20/A] and research contributing to this chapter was funded through the ethical, legal and social implications work package of the IMI European Prevention of Alzheimer's Dementia project.

References

Ankeny, R.A. and Leonelli, S. (2018) 'Organisms in experimental research', in M. Dietrich, M. Borrello and O. Harman (eds) *Handbook of the Historiography of Biology*, Cham: Springer International Publishing, pp 1–25.

Ankeny, R.A., Leonelli, S., Nelson, N.C. and Ramsden, E. (2014) 'Making organisms model human behavior: Situated models in North-American alcohol research, since 1950', *Science in Context*, 27(3): 485–509.

Ballenger, J. (2006) 'The biomedical deconstruction of senility and the persistent stigmatization of old age in the United States', in A. Leibing and L. Cohen (eds) *Thinking About Dementia: Culture, Loss, and the Anthropology of Senility*, New Brunswick, NJ: Rutgers University Press, pp 106–120.

BBC News (2022) 'Alzheimer's drug lecanemab hailed as momentous breakthrough', *BBC News*, 30 November. Available from: https://www.bbc.com/news/health-63749586 [Accessed 4 January 2023].

Beard, R.L. (2004) 'Advocating voice: Organisational, historical and social milieux of the Alzheimer's disease movement', *Sociology of Health & Illness*, 26(6): 797–819.

Beard, R.L. and Neary, T.M. (2013) 'Making sense of nonsense: Experiences of mild cognitive impairment', *Sociology of Health & Illness*, 35(1): 130–146.

Brown, N. (2000) 'Organising/disorganising the breakthrough motif: Dolly the cloned ewe meets Astrid the hybrid pig', in N. Brown, B. Rappert and A. Webster (eds) *Contested Futures: A Sociology of Prospective Techno-Science*, Aldershot: Ashgate, pp 87–108.

Bruno, A. and Lapsley, I. (2018) 'The emergence of an accounting practice: The fabrication of a government accrual accounting system', *Accounting, Auditing & Accountability Journal*, 31(4): 1045–1066.

Caron-Flinterman, J.F., Broerse, J.E.W. and Bunders, J.F.G. (2007) 'Patient partnership in decision-making on biomedical research: Changing the network', *Science, Technology, & Human Values*, 32(3): 339–368.

Cartwright, L. (1998) 'Community and the public body in breast cancer media activism', *Cultural Studies*, 12(2): 117–138.

Davies, G. (2010) 'Captivating behaviour: Mouse models, experimental genetics and reductionist returns in the neurosciences', *The Sociological Review*, 58(1): 53–72.

Davies, G. (2012) 'What is a humanized mouse? Remaking the species and spaces of translational medicine', *Body & Society*, 18(3–4): 126–155.

Davies, G. (2013a) 'Arguably big biology: Sociology, spatiality and the knockout mouse project', *BioSocieties*, 8(4): 417–431.

Davies, G. (2013b) 'Mobilizing experimental life: Spaces of becoming with mutant mice', *Theory, Culture & Society*, 30(7–8): 129–153.

Davies, G., Gorman, R. and Crudgington, B. (2020) 'Which patient takes centre stage? Placing patient voices in animal research', in S. Atkinson and R. Hunt (eds) *GeoHumanities and Health*, New York, NY: Springer, pp 141–155.

Davies, G., Gorman, R. and King, G. (2022) *Informing Involvement around Animal Research: Report and Resources from the Animal Research Nexus Project*. Available from: https://animalresearchnexus.org/publications/informing-involvement-around-animal-research [Accessed 21 April 2022].

Davies, G., Gorman, R. and King, G. (2024a) '"Knowledge is power, and I do want to know more": Exploring assumptions around patient involvement in animal research', in G. Davies, B. Greenhough, P. Hobson-West, R.W.G. Kirk, A. Palmer and E. Roe (eds) *Researching Animal Research*, Manchester: Manchester University Press, pp 265–289.

Davies, G., Greenhough, B., Hobson-West, P., Kirk, R.G.W., Palmer, A. and Roe, E. (eds) (2024b) *Researching Animal Research: What the Humanities and Social Sciences can Contribute to Laboratory Animal Science and Welfare*, Manchester: Manchester University Press.

Dietrich, M.R., Ankeny, R., Crowe, N., Green, S. and Leonelli, S. (2020) 'How to choose your research organism', *Studies in History and Philosophy of Science Part C: Studies in History and Philosophy of Biological and Biomedical Sciences*, 80: 101227.

Duff, K. (1999) 'Transgenic mouse models of Alzheimer's disease', in W.E. Crusio and R.T. Gerlai (eds) *Techniques in the Behavioral and Neural Sciences*, Oxford: Elsevier, pp 880–894.

Fox, P. (1989) 'From senility to Alzheimer's Disease: The rise of the Alzheimer's Disease movement', *The Milbank Quarterly*, 67(1): 58–102.

Gorman, R. and Davies, G. (2020) 'When "cultures of care" meet: Entanglements and accountabilities at the intersection of animal research and patient involvement in the UK', *Social & Cultural Geography*, 24(1): 121–139.

Götz, J. and Ittner, L.M. (2008) 'Animal models of Alzheimer's disease and frontotemporal dementia', *Nature Reviews Neuroscience*, 9(7): 532–544.

Gove, D., Diaz-Ponce, A., Georges, J., Moniz-Cook, E., Mountain, G., Chattat, R., et al (2018) 'Alzheimer Europe's position on involving people with dementia in research through PPI (patient and public involvement)', *Aging & Mental Health*, 22(6): 723–729.

Greenberg, B.D. (2012) 'Transcript of talks at the NIH Alzheimer's Disease summit 2012', *Alzheimer's Disease Research Summit 2012: Path to Treatment and Prevention*, Natcher Auditorium, NIH Campus, Bethesda, Maryland, National Institutes of Health. Available from: https://www.nia.nih.gov/sites/default/files/d7/alzheimers_summit_day_1_transcript.doc

Hampel, H., Au, R., Mattke, S., van der Flier, W., Aisen, P., Apostolova, L., et al (2022) 'Designing the next-generation clinical care pathway for Alzheimer's disease', *Nature Aging*, 2(8): 692–703.

Hardy, J. (2006) 'Alzheimer's disease: The amyloid cascade hypothesis: An update and reappraisal', *Journal of Alzheimer's Disease*, 9(s3): 151–153.

Hardy, J.A. and Higgins, G.A. (1992) 'Alzheimer's Disease: The amyloid cascade hypothesis', *Science*, 256(5054): 184–185.

Joseph, A. (2021) 'Q&A: The CEO of the Alzheimer's Association on the approval of Aduhelm – and why critics should stop dwelling on the decision', *STAT*, 16 June. Available from: https://www.statnews.com/2021/06/16/qa-ceo-alzheimers-association-on-aduhelm/ [Accessed 3 February 2023].

Katzman, R. and Bick, K. (2000) *Alzheimer Disease: The Changing View*, San Diego, CA: Academic Press.

Knorr-Cetina, K. (1981) *The Manufacture of Knowledge: An Essay on the Constructivist and Contextual Nature of Science*, Oxford: Pergamon Press.

Latour, B. and Woolgar, S. (1979) *Laboratory Life: The Construction of Scientific Facts*, Princeton, NJ: Princeton University Press.

Leonelli, S. (2012) 'When humans are the exception: Cross-species databases at the interface of biological and clinical research', *Social Studies of Science*, 42(2): 214–236.

Leonelli, S. and Ankeny, R.A. (2012) 'Re-thinking organisms: The impact of databases on model organism biology', *Studies in History and Philosophy of Science Part C: Studies in History and Philosophy of Biological and Biomedical Sciences*, 43(1): 29–36.

Maccarthy, J., Guerin, S., Wilson, A. and Dorris, E. (2019) 'Facilitating public and patient involvement in basic and preclinical health research', *PLoS ONE*, 14(5): 1–16.

Macleod, M. and the University of Edinburgh Research Strategy Group (2022) 'Improving the reproducibility and integrity of research: What can different stakeholders contribute?', *BMC Research Notes*, 15(146).

Marris, C. and Rose, N. (2010) 'Open engagement: Exploring public participation in the Biosciences', *PLOS Biology*, 8(11): e1000549.

Milne, R. (2018) 'From people with dementia to people with data: Participation and value in Alzheimer's Disease research', *BioSocieties*, 13(3): 1–17.

Milne, R. (2020) 'The rare and the common: scale and the genetic imaginary in Alzheimer's disease drug development', *New Genetics and Society*, 39(1): 101–126.

Milne, R. and Latimer, J. (2020) 'Alzheimer's disease and the development of a post-genomic science', *New Genetics and Society*, 39(1): 1–12.

Moreira, T. (2009) 'Testing promises: Truth and hope in drug development and evaluation in Alzheimer's disease', in J. Ballenger, P. Whitehouse, C. Lyketsos, P. Rabins, and J. Karlawish (eds) *Treating dementia: do we have a pill for it?*, Baltimore, MD: Johns Hopkins University Press.

Moreira, T. and Palladino, P. (2005) 'Between truth and hope: On Parkinson's disease, neurotransplantation and the production of the "self"', *History of the Human Sciences*, 18(3): 55–82.

Mullan, M., Crawford, F., Axelman, K., Houlden, H., Lilius, L., Winblad, B., et al (1992) 'A pathogenic mutation for probable Alzheimer's disease in the APP gene at the N–terminus of β–amyloid', *Nature Genetics*, 1(5): 345–347.

Nelson, N.C. (2018) *Model Behavior: Animal Experiments, Complexity, and the Genetics of Psychiatric Disorders*, Chicago, IL: University of Chicago Press.

Nilsberth, C., Westlind-Danielsson, A., Eckman, C., Condron, M., Axelman, K., Forsell, C., et al (2001) 'The "Arctic" APP mutation (E693G) causes Alzheimer's disease by enhanced Aβ protofibril formation', *Nature Neuroscience*, 4(9): 887–893.

Parry, B. (2020) 'Patents and the challenge of "open source" in an emergent biological commons or ... the strange case of Betty Crocker and the mouse', *BioSocieties*, 15(2): 294–315.

Pickett, J. and Murray, M. (2018) 'Editorial: Patient and public involvement in dementia research: Setting new standards', *Dementia*, 17(8): 939–943.

Preston, A.M., Cooper, D.J. and Coombs, R.W. (1992) 'Fabricating budgets: A study of the production of management budgeting in the national health service', *Accounting, Organizations and Society*, 17(6): 561–593.

Rader, K.A. (2004) *Making Mice: Standardizing Animals for American Biomedical Research, 1900–1955*, Princeton, NJ: Princeton University Press.

Rheinberger, H.-J. (1997) *Toward a History of Epistemic Things: Synthesizing Proteins in the Test Tube*, Stanford, CA: Stanford University Press.

Saunders, S., Ritchie, C., Russ, T., Muniz-Terrera, G. and Milne, R. (2022) 'Assessing and disclosing test results for "mild cognitive impairment": The perspective of old age psychiatrists in Scotland', *BMC Geriatrics*, 22(165).

Shared Learning Group on Involvement (2016) 'Involving people in laboratory based research: A discussion paper'. Available from: http://slginvolvement.org.uk/wp-content/uploads/2016/09/Lab-based-research-FINAL-10-8-16-public.pdf [Accessed 10 June 2019].

Vitek, M.P., Araujo, J., Fossel, M., Greenberg, B., Howell, G., Sukoff Rizzo, S., et al (2020) 'Translational animal models for Alzheimer's disease: An Alzheimer's Association Business Consortium Think Tank', *Alzheimer's & Dementia: Translational Research & Clinical Interventions*, 6(1): e12114.

Walsh, S., Merrick, R., Richard, E., Nurock, S. and Brayne, C. (2022) 'Lecanemab for Alzheimer's disease', *BMJ*, 379: o3010.

Wilson, P., Mathie, E., Keenan, J., McNeilly, E., Goodman, C., Howe, A., et al (2015) 'Research with patient and public involvement: A realist evaluation – the RAPPORT study', *Health Services and Delivery Research*, 3(38).

Woodard, J.S. (1966) 'Alzheimer's disease in late adult life', *The American Journal of Pathology*, 49(6): 1157–1169.

3

What we know about dementia in animals

Lorena Sordo

Introduction

Ageing is an inevitable part of life that is accompanied by important anatomical, biological and physiological changes. The onset and severity of these changes varies from person to person due to individual (for example, genetics) and external factors (for example, nutrition, exercise, lifestyle) that affect the way the different tissues and organs respond to the ageing process (Cotman et al, 2002; Glass et al, 2013; Melis et al, 2013).

The brain is highly vulnerable to the ageing process due to its high oxygen requirements and its limited ability to regenerate (Rink and Khanna, 2011). The deteriorating effect of ageing on the brain goes beyond modifying the gross morphology (shape) and vasculature (blood vessels) of the brain, as well as the structure and function of brain cells, as these changes trigger alterations in neurotransmitters and hormones which ultimately lead to the deterioration of cognitive abilities and dementia.

Dementia is a devastating disease that affects around 55 million people, worldwide, and its prevalence is expected to increase to 139 million people by 2050 (World Health Organization, 2022). Dementia is an umbrella term used to describe a range of symptoms, such as confusion, memory loss and language problems, among others. These symptoms can be caused by different diseases and/or conditions that affect distinct areas of the brain; therefore, there are different types of dementia, including frontotemporal dementia, vascular dementia, Lewy body dementia and Alzheimer's disease, and it is not unusual for individuals to present a combination of more than one type of dementia, also known as mixed dementia.

Alzheimer's disease (AD) is not only one of the many different types of dementia; AD is, in fact, the most common type and causes around two-thirds of all dementia cases (Laferla and Green, 2012). There are two forms of AD, familial and sporadic. Most cases of AD result from the sporadic form of the disease, with far fewer cases of the familial or genetic form (Laferla and Green, 2012); the two of them differ by the age of onset, the progression of disease and their cognitive symptoms (Laferla and Green, 2012; Ricciarelli and Fedele, 2017). Familial AD has a genetic origin due to mutations in the amyloid precursor protein (APP) (Levy et al, 1990; Goate et al, 1991) and presenilin 1 and 2 (St George-Hyslop et al, 1987; Levy-Lahad et al, 1995; Rogaev et al, 1995) (PS1 and PS2, respectively) genes that promote overproduction of amyloid-β (Aβ) (Hardy and Higgins, 1992). The cause of the sporadic form of AD, however, remains unclear. It has been proposed that this form of AD results from the abnormal accumulation of Aβ and tau in the brain. Both Aβ and tau are proteins that are naturally produced in the body and are involved in normal physiological functions. However, when they abnormally accumulate in the brain, they become toxic, promoting further aggregation and forming the characteristic Aβ plaques, and tau neurofibrillary tangles (NFT). Both Aβ plaques and NFT are the two major hallmarks of AD, and their abnormal deposition in the brain promotes dysfunction of neurons and synapses leading to neuronal death and cognitive impairment (Dekosky and Scheff, 1990; Terry et al, 1991).

For decades, animals have served as models for the study of different diseases. The use of animals in research has improved our understanding of human biology and physiology and has helped to unravel the causes and mechanism of action behind certain diseases, as well as helping us to develop new drugs and test the effectiveness and safety of treatments. Nonetheless, besides the ethical and animal welfare implications, using animals in research has several disadvantages. Since animals' anatomy, metabolism and physiology differ considerably to that in humans, translating findings from animals to humans may not necessarily reflect what would happen in the human body.

Over the last decades, mice have been one of the most commonly used animal models for the study of AD; however, mice do not naturally develop either AD or its associated neuropathology (that is, Aβ and NFT) (Laferla and Green, 2012; Volloch et al, 2020). For this reason, transgenic mice with specific genetic mutations have been developed to recreate the neuropathology of the disease (Laferla and Green, 2012). It is important to note that these mice models mimic the genetics of familial AD, instead of the sporadic form of the disease which, as mentioned previously, is the most common form of AD (Laferla and Green, 2012; Ricciarelli and Fedele, 2017). Since mutations on the APP gene that lead to abnormal Aβ production are known to exist in the familial form of AD, transgenic mice that overproduce APP were initially created. These mice develop cognitive decline and severe Aβ pathology which is, in fact, very similar to that seen in the human brain (Games et al, 1995; Hsiao et al, 1996; Sturchler-Pierrat et al, 1997; Laferla and Green, 2012; Volloch et al, 2020); however, this strain of mice does not form NFT (Laferla and Green, 2012). Hence, a double transgenic mouse model had to be developed that overexpressed APP and formed Aβ plaques, as well as developing NFT and cognitive deficits (Lewis et al, 2001; Schindowski et al, 2006; Laferla and Green, 2012). Since then, several strains of mice with single, double or multiple mutations in different genes have been created to mimic Aβ and tau pathologies. Even though these models have been shown to be useful in elucidating AD pathology, it has become clear that extrapolating findings from mice models to humans can be challenging due to natural differences between species (Laferla and Green, 2012). For instance, some of the drugs used in pre-clinical trials that have been successful in mice models, have been unsuccessful in clinical trials in people with AD. In the mice models, some of these drugs have been shown to reduce the production and aggregation of Aβ, while increasing its clearance from the brain and reversing cognitive damage; however, these positive outcomes were not observed in humans with AD (Volloch et al, 2020). Although this is only one example of unsuccessful translational research within a vast pool of successful ones, it is not unreasonable to question whether mice models are a good representation of human AD and/or whether there could be more accurate animal models (Ricciarelli and Fedele, 2017). Recently, other animals including dogs and cats have been shown to spontaneously produce the two hallmarks of AD (that is, Aβ and tau) and to develop an age-related cognitive decline, known as cognitive dysfunction syndrome, making them potential natural models.

In the first section of this chapter, we will describe the age-related behavioural and cognitive changes commonly seen in animals; whereas the AD-like neuropathology and other age-related brain changes will be covered in the second section.

Age-related behavioural and cognitive changes

Behavioural changes

Scientific advances in veterinary medicine and nutrition have significantly increased the life expectancy of pets. Recent studies have shown that the life expectancy of dogs and cats is around 12 and 14 years, respectively (O'Neill et al, 2015; Teng et al, 2022); although in dogs, ageing is highly breed-dependent. Consequently, it is not unreasonable to consider that long-lived animals may develop age-related changes similar to those observed in elderly individuals with cognitive impairment and, particularly, with AD.

Cognitive dysfunction syndrome (CDS) is the term given to the age-related decline in cognitive functions of aged dogs and cats that cannot be attributed to other medical conditions. CDS is a highly prevalent condition that affects 68 per cent of dogs (Neilson et al, 2001) and 50 per cent of cats (Moffat and Landsberg, 2003) over 15 years of age; with the early signs appearing around 11 years of age for both (Neilson et al, 2001; Moffat and Landsberg, 2003).

Dogs with CDS display behavioural changes that are summarised by the acronym DISHAAL, which stands for *D*isorientation; changes in *I*nteractions with their owners and other pets in the household; *S*leep-wake cycles alterations; *H*ouse-soiling; changes in *A*ctivity levels; *A*nxiety; and deficits in *L*earning and memory (Landsberg et al, 2003; 2012). Cats display many of these behaviours listed, however, the most frequent one in this species is excessive vocalisation, which is not included in DISHAAL. For this reason, behavioural changes in cats have the acronym VISHDAAL, which summarises the common abnormal behaviours in aged cats, ordered by prevalence (Sordo and Gunn-Moore, 2021). VISHDAAL refers to increased *V*ocalisation, which are more frequent at night; changes in *I*nteractions (that is, becoming more affectionate and demanding of attention as well as less tolerant to other animals); altered *S*leep-wake cycles; *H*ouse-soiling; *D*isorientation in space (for example, forgetting where the food bowl is) and/or in time (for example, forgetting if they have eaten); altered *A*ctivity levels (for example, aimless wandering); *A*nxiety; and memory and *L*earning deficits. Despite being the most obvious and frequent behavioural change in cats with CDS, the cause of the increased vocalisation remains unclear. In a questionnaire-based study, owners of cats with CDS were asked what they thought to be the likely cause for their cat's increased vocalisation, with most of the owners reporting disorientation (41 per cent) and seeking for attention (41 per cent) as the most likely causes, followed by looking for resources, such as water or food (16 per cent) and, finally, pain (3 per cent) (Černá et al, 2020).

Since CDS is a highly frequent condition in aged dogs and cats, it is not unreasonable to ponder whether other elderly animals may experience it as well. Anecdotal evidence suggests that aged horses also display abnormal behaviours, such as disorientation in familiar places, aimless wandering and difficulty recognising familiar objects, among others; however, to date, CDS has not been systematically characterised in horses. Further research is needed to identify age-related behavioural changes and their prevalence in equines.

Cognitive impairment

The term cognition refers to the mental processes or integration that occur in the brain such as thinking, memory, attention, perception and learning. In humans, cognition can be measured using a battery of tests that evaluate thinking, memory and problem-solving skills. Furthermore, these tests help to understand and determine whether an individual may be developing cognitive decline. The Mini-Mental State Examination is a commonly used test that assesses orientation, registration, short-term memory and language, by asking specific questions (for example, what is the year/day?), to name and recall objects, to count and do mental calculations, to follow commands, as well as reading, writing, copying and drawing. Since animals are unable to answer questions and to complete these same tasks, adaptations of the tests have been developed to assess cognitive functions in animals. Even though the tasks are not the same, these tests aim to assess the same cognitive domains.

In dogs, the use of standardised cognitive tests is frequently limited to laboratory settings. Elderly dogs develop age-related cognitive decline in domains such as learning, memory and executive function. Tasks that measure function of the prefrontal cortex, such as visuospatial working memory and reversal memory, have shown to be highly sensitive to ageing (Head et al, 1998; Tapp et al, 2003; Studzinski et al, 2006). Impairments in these tasks as well as in those assessing short-term working memory are believed to occur as early as six years of age (Studzinski et al, 2006). In contrast, tasks that do not rely on prefrontal function, such as allocentric and egocentric visuospatial learning, may be affected later (Milgram et al, 1999; 2002; Colle et al, 2000; Christie et al, 2005). Furthermore, aged dogs have shown poor performance when solving tasks associated with greater memory demand, such as the non-matching to position test, that assesses spatial memory (Head et al, 1995; Studzinski et al, 2006) and has also been useful to detect early memory decline (Studzinski et al, 2006).

Aged dogs have also shown deficits in learning tasks that require using visual stimuli, such as spatial learning (Christie et al, 2005), size concept learning (Tapp et al, 2003), size discrimination learning (Head et al, 1998; Tapp et al, 2003) and object recognition (Milgram et al, 1994). Since sensory decline is a frequent consequence of canine ageing (Landsberg and Araujo, 2005), it can be argued that aged dogs may perform worse in these tasks due to impaired vision. Nonetheless, aged dogs have also shown to perform well when they can use visual cues to complete a task, such as simple visual discrimination, suggesting that poor performance in these tasks is not associated with age-related sensory deficits (Milgram et al, 1994; Head et al, 1997).

In many of the neuropsychological tests mentioned earlier, there has been a great variability in cognitive scores between individual dogs. While some aged dogs displayed a marked cognitive decline, others performed as well as younger dogs (Adams et al, 2000). This individual variability has also been described in humans (Serrano-Pozo et al, 2011a), rodents (Markowska et al, 1989) and non-human primates (Rapp and Amaral, 1991; Rapp, 1993). Interestingly, poor cognitive performance in dogs has been linked to the presence of neuropathology, particularly with the extent of Aβ deposition in the brain (Head et al, 1998), which highlights the importance of combining cognitive test scoring with neuropathological findings to establish if any correlation exists that may reflect poor cognition.

In cats, a few laboratory-based studies have shown that cognition starts deteriorating at around ten years of age (Harrison and Buchwald, 1982; 1983; Levine et al, 1987a), with elderly cats showing an age-dependent decline in reversal learning and discrimination tasks (Cotman and Head, 2008; Milgram et al, 2011). It is important to highlight that testing cognition in cats can be challenging, especially as cats are not as motivated by food as dogs are (Gunn-Moore et al, 2007; Landsberg et al, 2012). Furthermore, elderly cats become highly sensitive to changes in their environment (Houpt and Beaver, 1981), which may affect their performance in cognitive testing.

With most of the canine and feline cognition studied in laboratory settings, assessing age-related cognitive decline in pet dogs and cats may be more relevant as they share the same environment as humans, and they benefit from social, intellectual and environmental enrichment. Simple tasks such as the open field test and the mirror test are also sensitive to ageing and can be used in non-laboratory settings (Head and Milgram, 1992; Milgram et al, 1994). In the open field test, aged dogs showed less interest when presented with novel objects and a reduced exploratory behaviour; whereas younger dogs tended to explore and engage more (Siwak et al, 2001). In the mirror test, however, older dogs interacted more with their own reflections, suggesting a lack of recognition of self, which is also a common sign that frequently occurs at severe stages of AD in humans (Siwak et al, 2001).

The use of owner-reported questionnaires is another efficient way to assess behavioural changes and cognition in pets in at-home settings. Currently, there are two validated questionnaires that are sensitive to behavioural and cognitive ageing in dogs (Salvin et al, 2011; Madari et al, 2015). These questionnaires assess relevant areas of behaviour and cognition by measuring the frequency of abnormal behaviours (that is, DISHAAL), and have proven to be a successful aid in the diagnosis of CDS, as well as determining severity and progression of disease in dogs. These same questionnaires are also used for the diagnosis of CDS in cats, as clinical metrology instruments are yet to be developed for this species.

The evidence covered in this section demonstrates that elderly animals experience age-related brain changes that lead to abnormal behaviours and cognitive decline. Given that animals affected by CDS experience a reduced responsiveness to stimuli, altered awareness, and learning and memory deficits, among others, CDS in animals has been compared to mild cognitive impairment and AD in humans.

AD-like neuropathology and other age-related brain changes

Ageing not only leads to behavioural and cognitive changes in animals, as evidence demonstrates that some animals develop the neuropathological changes commonly seen in the AD brain (that is, Aβ and tau deposition), as well as other age-related brain changes including brain atrophy and neuronal loss, among others.

Amyloid-β pathology

As mentioned previously, the Aβ protein derives from the APP, a protein found in the cells of different tissues, including the brain (Hardy and Allsop, 1991; Perl, 2010; Ricciarelli and Fedele, 2017). The APP protein is cleaved, at different sites, by three enzymes: alpha (α), beta (β) and gamma (γ)-secretases. Depending on the site that it is cleaved, this process can lead to one of two pathways: the non-amyloidogenic pathway, which does not generate Aβ; and the amyloidogenic pathway, in which Aβ is generated (Volloch et al, 2020) and which will be discussed in this section.

In the amyloidogenic pathway, APP is cleaved by β- and γ-secretases, releasing Aβ into the brain parenchyma (extracellular space), where it may accumulate (Hardy and Higgins, 1992; Perl, 2010). Since the second cleavage can occur at multiple sites, various lengths of Aβ can be generated (Volloch et al, 2020); the most common forms of Aβ in AD contain either 40 or 42 amino acids (Aβ40 and Aβ42, respectively) (Ricciarelli and Fedele, 2017). Aβ40 is the most abundant form and accumulates within the walls of capillaries in the brain, known as cerebral amyloid angiopathy (CAA) (Selkoe et al, 1987; Selkoe, 1997; Perl, 2010; Volloch et al, 2020); whereas Aβ42 aggregates and form senile plaques (Perl, 2010) (Figure 3.1). The formation of these senile plaques initiates when the Aβ fragments located in the parenchyma aggregate and form small clusters known as oligomers; bundles of oligomers form fibrils which may further aggregate and form β-sheets, leading to the formation of the characteristic senile plaques (Perl, 2010; Volloch et al, 2020).

The amyloid cascade hypothesis proposes that the aggregation of Aβ plaques triggers a series of processes, including neuroinflammation and neurotoxicity, promoting hyperphosphorylation of tau and formation of NFT, leading to neuronal dysfunction and cognitive impairment (Hardy and Higgins, 1992; Dickson et al, 1995). However, there is controversy in

Figure 3.1: Amyloid-β (Aβ) pathology in the Alzheimer's disease brain. Senile plaques have a core centre and are predominantly made of Aβ42 (left); whereas cerebral amyloid angiopathy (CAA) mostly contains Aβ40 which accumulates within blood vessel walls (right).

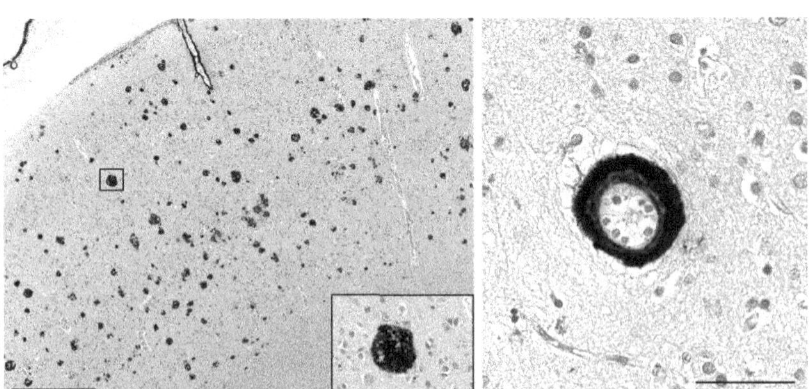

Source: Images used with permission from Professor Elizabeth Head

Figure 3.2: Amyloid-β (Aβ) senile plaques (left) and cerebral amyloid angiopathy (CAA; right) in the dog brain

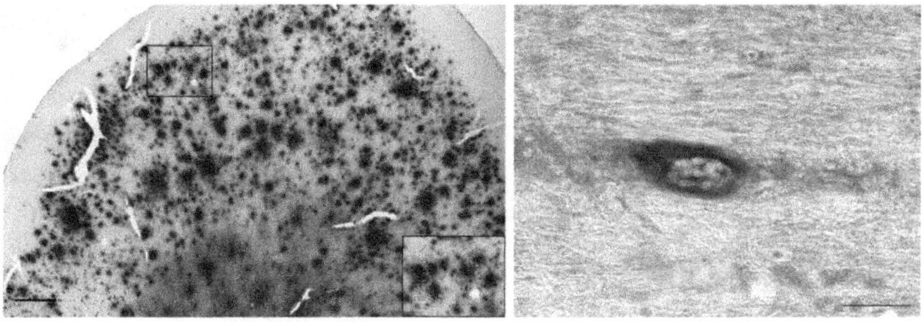

Source: Images used with permission from Professor Elizabeth Head

the field around this hypothesis. In humans, Aβ starts accumulating as early as 20 years of age (Gonneaud et al, 2017). Even though Aβ deposition may start decades before clinical signs appear, senile plaques have also been found in the brains of elderly individuals with no clinical signs of dementia (Selkoe et al, 1987), suggesting that the presence of Aβ senile plaques might not necessarily be the initiator of these mechanisms.

In dogs, Aβ plaques start accumulating in the prefrontal cortex around the age of nine years (Head et al, 2000) (Figure 3.2). Unsurprisingly, the development of Aβ plaques in dogs is breed-dependent, with some breeds developing them earlier than others (Bobik et al, 1994; Head et al, 2000). While the presence of Aβ plaques has been described in clinically normal dogs, it has been suggested that the appearance of cognitive deficits likely reflects progression and severity of Aβ pathology (Cummings et al, 1996a; Head et al, 1998; Colle et al, 2000). For example, in a study that assessed age-related cognitive changes in laboratory beagles, those with Aβ plaques in the prefrontal cortex performed poorer in tasks measuring executive function (Head et al, 1998).

The progression of Aβ pathology in dogs is also similar to that seen in humans. After the first Aβ deposits appear in the canine prefrontal cortex, the pathology progresses to the entorhinal and parietal cortices, reaching the occipital cortex at later stages of disease (Head et al, 2000). This pattern is consistent with that reported in the aged human brain, in which the frontal cortex is also affected earlier (Selkoe et al, 1987; Braak and Braak, 1991; Ishihara et al, 1991; Head et al, 2000; Thal et al, 2002). This is not surprising given that the amino acid sequence of Aβ in dogs is almost identical to that in human Aβ (Uniprot Consortium, 2023) and, for this reason, the dog has been considered to be a good model for neurodegenerative diseases and for therapeutic interventions that target Aβ (Selkoe et al, 1987; Head et al, 2008).

Besides Aβ senile plaques, dogs also accumulate CAA (Selkoe et al, 1987; Uchida et al, 1990; 1991; Colle et al, 2000), which has been associated with

Figure 3.3: Diffuse amyloid-β (Aβ) deposits (left) and cerebral amyloid angiopathy (CAA; right) in the brain of a cat with CDS

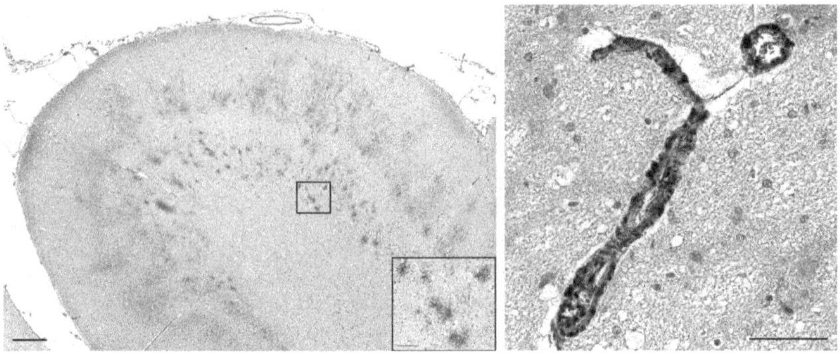

cognitive impairment and brain haemorrhages (Uchida et al, 1990; Colle et al, 2000). Virtually all the dogs over 13 years of age may display CAA, particularly in the occipital cortex (Wegiel et al, 1995). Similarly, in humans with AD, CAA is a frequent neuropathological finding in the occipital and parietal cortices, with its accumulation resulting in weakening of the capillary wall that leads to rupture and micro-haemorrhages (Revesz et al, 2002; 2003).

Aβ pathology and CAA have also been described in cats over ten years of age (Cummings et al, 1996c; Nakamura et al, 1996; Brellou et al, 2005; Head et al, 2005; Gunn-Moore et al, 2006) (Figure 3.3). Even though the amino acid sequence of Aβ in cats is 96.8 per cent similar to human Aβ (Uniprot Consortium, 2023), cats do not form senile plaques, but rather accumulate Aβ in a diffuse pattern (Cummings et al, 1996c; Nakamura et al, 1996; Head et al, 2005; Gunn-Moore et al, 2006; 2007; Chambers et al, 2015; Sordo et al, 2021). Diffuse Aβ deposits, however, are not unique to the feline brain. In humans, diffuse Aβ deposits are believed to be an early stage of the Aβ senile plaques (Hardy and Allsop, 1991; Perl, 2010). These diffuse deposits contain few to no fibrils and have been reported in the brains of elderly individuals with no signs of cognitive impairment (Hardy and Allsop, 1991; Perl, 2010).

The pattern and distribution of Aβ in cats is similar to that in humans with AD, with Aβ aggregation occurring in cortical areas during early stages of disease that later progresses to other areas such as the hippocampus and, finally, the cerebellum (Sordo et al, 2021). Unlike Aβ pathology in dogs, whether Aβ pathology correlates with cognitive impairment in cats remains unclear. While some studies have found that cats with Aβ pathology display signs of CDS, particularly excessive vocalisation, confusion and aimless wandering (Cummings et al, 1996c; Gunn-Moore et al, 2006), other studies have found no association between them (Head et al, 2005; Sordo et al, 2021).

Aβ pathology has also been observed in non-human primates, including cynomolgus monkeys (Nakamura et al, 1995; Oikawa et al, 2010), orangutans

(Selkoe et al, 1987), gorillas (Kimura et al, 2001), chimpanzees (Rosen et al, 2008), rhesus macaques (Poduri et al, 1994), baboons (Schultz et al, 2000a; 2000b), squirrel monkeys (Chambers et al, 2010), common marmosets (Geula et al, 2002) and mouse lemurs (Bons et al, 1992), among others, and in other aged mammals such as equines (that is, horses [Jahns et al, 2006; Capucchio et al, 2010] and donkeys [Malbon et al, 2022]), sheep (Braak et al, 1994; Nelson et al, 1994; Reid et al, 2017), degus (Tarragon et al, 2013), wolverines (Roertgen et al, 1996), polar bears (Johnstone et al, 1991; Tekirian et al, 1996), leopards (Chambers et al, 2012), cheetahs (Serizawa et al, 2012) and dolphins (Gunn-Moore et al, 2018; Vacher et al, 2022). Notably, besides dogs and cats, CAA has also been reported in gorillas (Márquez et al, 2008) and cynomolgus monkeys (Nakamura et al, 1995).

It is clear that Aβ pathology is a common age-related neuropathological finding in several species; however, further studies are needed to better understand its association with cognitive decline in animals.

Tau pathology

Tau is a protein located in the body and axons of neurons that provides stability and maintains structure (Lee et al, 2005; Perl, 2010; Kametani and Hasegawa, 2018). Under physiological conditions, tau can undergo phosphorylation and dephosphorylation processes in order to complete its normal functions. However, pathological conditions may promote excessive phosphorylation (hyperphosphorylation) of this protein. When abnormally hyperphosphorylated, tau aggregates within neuronal bodies and forms NFT leading to neuronal death and neurodegeneration (Goedert et al, 1989; Hardy and Allsop, 1991; Lee et al, 2005; Perl, 2010) (Figure 3.4).

Figure 3.4: Neurofibrillary tangles (NFT) in human brain (left) and cat brain (right)

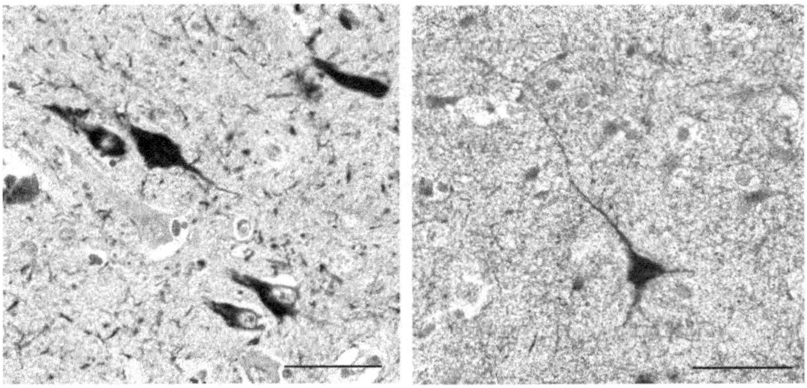

Source: Left image used with permission from Professor Elizabeth Head

In contrast to Aβ pathology, not many animals have shown to develop NFT. In fact, dogs were thought to be spared of tau pathology (Cummings et al, 1996b), until recent studies demonstrated the presence of abnormal tau aggregates in the canine brain, particularly in those with CDS (Schmidt et al, 2015; Smolek et al, 2016; Abey et al, 2021). As mentioned earlier, under physiological conditions, tau functions are regulated by the phosphorylation of amino acid residues (that is, serine, threonine and tyrosine) located at different domains within the sequence of tau. In humans, there are over 85 phosphorylation sites throughout the tau protein; these phosphorylation sites or epitopes can be recognised by specific antibodies commonly used in human neuropathological studies. For instance, the AT8 clone is the standard antibody used when assessing tau pathology, particularly in AD, which recognises the tau protein when phosphorylated at both Serine 202 and Threonine 205. Most of the studies in dogs have used the AT8 clone antibody and have been unsuccessful in detecting NFT in this species; however, in a recent study, tau labelling was identified in the brains of aged dogs using an antibody that binds to the Serine 396 residue (Abey et al, 2021); this epitope phosphorylates earlier than Serine 202 and Threonine 205 (that is, AT8 clone antibody), hence, recognising earlier stages of NFT (Augustinack et al, 2002; Mondragón-Rodríguez et al, 2014).

Similarly, for years, the presence of NFT in aged cats could not be determined. Even though cats produce similar isoforms to human tau (Head et al, 2005; Gunn-Moore et al, 2006; Chambers et al, 2015), earlier studies found no evidence of NFT in this species (Nakamura et al, 1996; Kuroki et al, 1997). In contrast, more recent studies have shown not only neuronal positive immunostaining for hyperphosphorylated tau (Head et al, 2005; Gunn-Moore et al, 2006), but also pre-tangles (that is, early stages of NFT [Chambers et al, 2015; Sordo et al, 2021]) which have been associated with CDS (Sordo et al, 2021) (Figure 3.4).

These findings suggest that pre-tangles in both dogs and cats rarely progress into fully mature NFT due to the animals' short lifespans; however, it is also plausible that the tau protein in these two species phosphorylates in different epitopes than human tau.

Notably, early NFT or pre-tangles are not exclusively found in dogs and cats, as these have been reported in cynomolgus monkeys (Nakamura et al, 1995; Oikawa et al, 2010), leopards (Chambers et al, 2012), cheetahs (Serizawa et al, 2012), brown bears (Cork et al, 1988), wolverines (Roertgen et al, 1996), degus (Tarragon et al, 2013), donkeys (Malbon et al, 2022) and dolphins (Gunn-Moore et al, 2018; Vacher et al, 2022). Furthermore, the presence of positive immunostaining for hyperphosphorylated tau has been reported in non-human primates such as chimpanzees (Rosen et al, 2008), mouse lemurs (Bons et al, 1992) and baboons (Schultz et al, 2000a; 2000b); and in other aged animals such as sheep (Braak et al, 1994; Nelson et al,

1994; Reid et al, 2017), goats (Braak et al, 1994) and horses (Capucchio et al, 2010). Of note, it is important to highlight the possibility that tau may also phosphorylate at different epitopes in these and other species.

Besides abnormal protein deposition, other age-related changes may negatively impact the anatomy and physiology of the brain leading to deterioration of cognition, such as brain atrophy and vascular changes.

Age-related brain changes in animals

Neuronal loss and brain atrophy

Neuronal loss is a frequent consequence of ageing that can be induced by disturbances in neuronal functions, such as alterations in autophagy (that is, the degradation of cell components), mitochondrial dysfunction, disturbances in the endoplasmic reticulum functions (that is, endoplasmic reticulum stress) or alterations in the ubiquitin system (Ghavami et al, 2014). Even though neuronal loss and reduced neurogenesis (that is, the process of formation of new neurons) frequently occur as a normal part of ageing, these have shown to be more severe in individuals with AD (West, 1993; Bobinski et al, 1997; Šimić et al, 1997). For example, the loss of cholinergic and hippocampal neurons are frequent findings in AD that are believed to impair cognition (Bartus et al, 1982; Coyle et al, 1983; Muir, 1997; Nelson et al, 2011). Eventually, significant neuronal loss leads to reduced neuronal density and, therefore, to brain atrophy.

Brain atrophy is characterised by a reduced brain size, alongside widened sulci, narrow gyri and thick meninges, and is one of the most remarkable age-related changes. In fact, the volume and weight of the brain declines at a rate of between 2 and 5 per cent per decade, starting at the age of 40 (Miller et al, 1980; Svennerholm et al, 1997). In AD, brain atrophy is known to frequently affect the frontal, parietal and temporal lobes, as well as the hippocampus (Kaye et al, 1997; Csernansky et al, 2005; Den Heijer et al, 2006; Morris et al, 2009; Martin et al, 2011). Consequently, this generalised cerebral atrophy results in enlargement of the ventricles (the interconnected chambers within the brain that are filled with cerebrospinal fluid) (Raz et al, 1997; Anderton, 2002; Barnes, 2003; Raz, 2004; Jack et al, 2005). Notably, some of these changes may appear decades before a clinical diagnosis of AD is made; therefore, these changes can be useful predictors and biomarkers of early stages of disease (Fox et al, 1996; Kaye et al, 1997; Den Heijer et al, 2006; Dickerson et al, 2011; Martin et al, 2011).

Neuronal loss has also been reported in canines. In aged dogs, hippocampal neurogenesis has been shown to decline up to 95 per cent (Hwang et al, 2007; Siwak-Tapp et al, 2007; Pekcec et al, 2008). Moreover, age-related neuronal loss may occur in various regions of the canine brain, such as the hippocampus, the Purkinje cells of the cerebellum, and the noradrenergic neurons in the locus coeruleus, and has been correlated with cognitive impairment and learning difficulties (Pugliese et al, 2007; Siwak-Tapp et al, 2008; Insua et al, 2010).

Anatomical age-related changes have also been described in dogs that primarily affect the frontal lobe and the hippocampus, and result in increased size of the ventricles (Vite et al, 1997; Su et al, 1998; Tapp et al, 2004b; Pugliese et al, 2010). As seen in humans, some of these changes occur earlier than others. For instance, atrophy of the frontal lobe may start in dogs as young as eight years old, progressing over time to a total brain atrophy starting by the age of 12 years (Fox, 1971; Tapp et al, 2004b); whereas hippocampal atrophy occurs after 11 years of age (Tapp et al, 2004a). Furthermore, recent studies have discovered an age-related significant reduction of the thickness of the interthalamic adhesion, a structure that connects both thalami, that has proven to be a useful *in vivo* method for the diagnosis of brain atrophy in dogs, particularly in those with CDS (Hasegawa et al, 2005; Noh et al, 2017).

Initial age-related changes, such as neuronal and synaptic loss, may start in the caudate nucleus of cats as young as seven years old and progress to more severe stages after the age of ten, causing motor function impairments (Levine et al, 1986; 1987b; 1987c; 1988). Furthermore, a reduced number of cholinergic and hippocampal neurons, as well as Purkinje cells, are known to occur in cats aged between 12 and 15 years old (Zhang et al, 2005; 2006; Chambers et al, 2015). It is not unreasonable to presume that these changes are likely to be more severe in cats with CDS; however, the aforementioned studies focused on understanding the histopathological changes associated with ageing and none of them included cats with a diagnosis of CDS in their study populations.

Similar to humans and dogs, age-related total brain atrophy, enlargement of the ventricles and a reduced interthalamic adhesion thickness have also been reported in cats (Babicsak et al, 2018a; 2018b). Nonetheless, the onset and progression of these anatomical changes, as well as their association with cognition in cats, remains unknown.

Vascular pathology

Besides CAA (described earlier) there are other vascular lesions, such as atherosclerosis and arteriolosclerosis, that are highly prevalent in AD and have been associated with cognitive impairment (Hofman et al, 1997; Van Oijen et al, 2007; Blevins et al, 2021). Atherosclerosis is the thickening of arteries caused by accumulation of fat and cholesterol within the artery walls. While this is a relatively common neuropathology in AD, it is a rare finding in animals.

Arteriolosclerosis is also highly prevalent in AD and is characterised by the thickening of blood vessel walls with a consequent narrowing of the lumen. In animals, arteriolosclerosis has been mostly described in horses (Capucchio et al, 2010). Notably, it has been reported that elderly cats can develop arteriolosclerosis as well, however, the pathology in this species is of the non-lipid variety (Landsberg and Araujo, 2005).

Vascular mineralisation is the abnormal deposition of minerals in the vascular system. Even though vascular mineralisation or calcification is another common age-related change, its clinical significance and involvement in the development of disease remains unknown. Mineralisation is known to occur in non-human primates (Yanai et al, 1994b), mice (Yanai et al, 1987), rats (Yanai et al, 1993), dogs (Fankhauser et al, 1965), cats (Mandara, 2003), horses (Capucchio et al, 2010; Martínez et al, 2012) and cows (Yanai et al, 1994a).

Of note, the association between these age-related vascular changes and cognition in animals remains undetermined and research is warranted.

Glial reactivity

Glial cells, such as microglia and astrocytes, are the most abundant non-neuronal cell types in the brain, which play a crucial role in maintaining brain homeostasis. Some of their functions include supporting neuronal function, promoting synaptic connections, transporting nutrients to neurons and clearing 'debris' from the brain, among others. Furthermore, both microglia and astrocytes are the brain response to injury and inflammation and their presence, in their reactive form, is a common finding in the AD brain and in other neurodegenerative diseases. Specifically, in AD, both reactive astrocytes and microglia are known to cluster around Aβ plaques, in order to clear them from the brain. In addition, their activity significantly increases when tau pathology is present (Serrano-Pozo et al, 2011b).

In animals, the presence of reactive astrocytes has been described in the white matter of aged dogs (Vite and Head, 2014) and horses (Capucchio et al, 2010). Interestingly, even though gliosis has been described in different cortical areas of cats with feline immunodeficiency virus (Abramo et al, 1995), there are no reports of age-related glial reactivity in the cat brain.

Conclusion

Ageing affects all living organisms in very similar ways, from alterations in molecular mechanisms to major pathological processes that lead to neurodegeneration and dementia. The evidence presented in this chapter reminds us that it is impossible to look into AD without referring to cognitive decline and/or dementia in animals, and vice versa. These interspecies similarities provide a unique opportunity to implement multidisciplinary approaches to better our understanding about ageing, cognitive decline and dementia. On the one hand, veterinarians may work alongside pet owners to compile questionnaires to determine early behavioural changes, whereas geriatricians and neurologists may help to adapt current human neuropsychological tests for their use in different animals. On the other hand, sociologists may examine potential risk factors, plus determine the impact of dementia in humans and animals, when they are the ones affected by it or when it affects someone they know (that is, friends or family) and/or their pets. While these are only a couple of examples of combined efforts across disciplines, it is clear that extrapolating findings from spontaneously occurring models may prove beneficial to increase our understanding about human and animal ageing processes, as well as to recognise early physiological and pathological age-related changes, and to facilitate interventions that can improve the quality of life of human and animal elder populations.

Acknowledgements

The author would like to thank Professor Elizabeth Head for sharing slides of AD neuropathology in humans and dogs for the present chapter. Professor Head's work was funded by NIH/NIA P30AG066519 and AG031764.

References

Abey, A., Davies, D., Goldsbury, C., Buckland, M., Valenzuela, M. and Duncan, T. (2021) 'Distribution of tau hyperphosphorylation in canine dementia resembles early Alzheimer's disease and other tauopathies', *Brain Pathology,* 31(1): 144–162.

Abramo, F., Bo, S., Canese, M.G. and Poli, A. (1995) 'Regional distribution of lesions in the central nervous system of cats infected with feline immunodeficiency virus', *AIDS Research and Human Retroviruses,* 11(10): 1247–1253.

Adams, B., Chan, A., Callahan, H. and Milgram, N.W. (2000) 'The canine as a model of human cognitive aging: Recent developments', *Progress in Neuro-Psychopharmacology and Biological Psychiatry,* 24(5): 675–692.

Anderton, B. (2002) 'Ageing of the brain', *Mechanisms of Ageing and Development,* 123(7): 811–817.

Augustinack, J.C., Schneider, A., Mandelkow, E.M. and Hyman, B.T. (2002) 'Specific tau phosphorylation sites correlate with severity of neuronal cytopathology in Alzheimer's disease', *Acta Neuropathologica,* 103(1): 26–35.

Babicsak, V.R., Klein, A.V., Tsunemi, M.H. and Vulcano, L.C. (2018a) 'Age-related changes of the cerebral ventricles of healthy domestic cats', *Pesquisa Veterinaria Brasileira,* 38(10): 1935–1941.

Babicsak, V.R., Klein, A.V., Tsunemi, M.H. and Vulcano, L.C. (2018b) 'Brain parenchymal changes during normal aging in domestic cats', *Pesquisa Veterinaria Brasileira,* 38(6): 1196–1202.

Barnes, C. (2003) 'Long-term potentiation and the ageing', *Philosophical Transactions of the Royal Society of London. Series B, Biological Sciences*, 358(1432): 765–772.

Bartus, R.T., Dean, R.L., Beer, B. and Lippa, A. S. (1982) 'The cholinergic hypothesis of geriatric memory dysfunction', *Science*, 217(4558): 408–417.

Blevins, B.L., Vinters, H.V., Love, S., Wilcock, D.M., Grinberg, L.T., Schneider, J., et al (2021) 'Brain arteriolosclerosis', *Acta Neuropathologica*, 141(1): 1–24.

Bobik, M., Thompson, T. and Russell, M. (1994) 'Amyloid deposition in various breeds of dogs', *Abstracts in Neuroscience*, 20: 172.

Bobinski, M., Wegiel, J., Tarnawski, M., Bobinski, M., Reisberg, B., De Leon, M.J., et al (1997) 'Relationships between regional neuronal loss and neurofibrillary changes in the hippocampal formation and duration and severity of Alzheimer disease', *Journal of Neuropathology & Experimental Neurology*, 56(4): 414–420.

Bons, N., Mestre, N. and Petter, A. (1992) 'Senile plaques and neurofibrillary changes in the brain of an aged lemurian primate, Microcebus murinus', *Neurobiology of Aging*, 13(1): 99–105.

Braak, H. and Braak, E. (1991) 'Neuropathological stageing of Alzheimer-related changes', *Acta Neuropathologica*, 82(4): 239–259.

Braak, H., Braak, E. and Strothjohann, M. (1994) 'Abnormally phosphorylated tau protein related to the formation of neurofibrillary tangles and neuropil threads in the cerebral cortex of sheep and goat', *Neuroscience Letters*, 171(1–2): 1–4.

Brellou, G., Vlemmas, I., Lekkas, S. and Papaioannou, N. (2005) 'Immunohistochemical investigation of amyloid beta-protein (Abeta) in the brain of aged cats', *Histology and Histopathology*, 20(3): 725–731.

Capucchio, M.T., Márquez, M., Pregel, P., Foradada, L., Bravo, M., Mattutino, G., et al (2010) 'Parenchymal and vascular lesions in ageing equine brains: Histological and immunohistochemical studies', *Journal of Comparative Pathology*, 142(1): 61–73.

Černá, P., Gardiner, H., Sordo, L., Tørnqvist-Johnsen, C. and Gunn-Moore, D.A. (2020) 'Potential causes of increased vocalisation in elderly cats with cognitive dysfunction syndrome as assessed by their owners', *Animals (Basel)*, 10(6): 1092.

Chambers, J.K., Kuribayashi, H., Ikeda, S.-I. and Une, Y. (2010) 'Distribution of neprilysin and deposit patterns of Aβ subtypes in the brains of aged squirrel monkeys (Saimiri sciureus)', *Amyloid*, 17(2): 75–82.

Chambers, J.K., Uchida, K., Harada, T., Tsuboi, M., Sato, M., Kubo, M., et al (2012) 'Neurofibrillary tangles and the deposition of a beta amyloid peptide with a novel N-Terminal epitope in the brains of wild tsushima leopard cats', *PLoS One*, 7(10): e46452.

Chambers, J.K., Tokuda, T., Uchida, K., Ishii, R., Tatebe, H., Takahashi, E., et al (2015) 'The domestic cat as a natural animal model of Alzheimer's disease', *Acta Neuropathologica Communications*, 3: 78.

Christie, L.-A., Studzinski, C.M., Araujo, J.A., Leung, C.S., Ikeda-douglas, C.J., Head, E., et al (2005) 'A comparison of egocentric and allocentric age-dependent spatial learning in the beagle dog', *Progress in Neuro-Psychopharmacology and Biological Psychiatry*, 29(3): 361–369.

Colle, M.-A., Hauw, J.-J., Crespeau, F., Uchihara, T., Akiyama, H., Checler, F., et al (2000) 'Vascular and parenchymal Aβ deposition in the aging dog: correlation with behavior', *Neurobiology of Aging*, 21(5): 695–704.

Cork, L.C., Powers, R.E., Selkoe, D.J., Davies, P., Geyer, J.J. and Price, D.L. (1988) 'Neurofibrillary tangles and senile plaques in aged bears', *Journal of Neuropathology & Experimental Neurology*, 47(6): 629–641.

Cotman, C.W. and Head, E. (2008) 'The canine (dog) model of human aging and disease: Dietary, environmental and immunotherapy approaches', *Journal of Alzheimer's Disease*, 15(4): 685–707.

Cotman, C.W., Head, E., Muggenburg, B.A., Zicker, S. and Milgram, N.W. (2002) 'Brain aging in the canine: A diet enriched in antioxidants reduces cognitive dysfunction', *Neurobiology of Aging*, 23(5): 809–818.

Coyle, J.T., Price, D.L. and Delong, M.R. (1983) 'Alzheimer's disease: A disorder of cortical cholinergic innervation', *Science*, 219(4589): 1184–1190.

Csernansky, J.G., Wang, L., Swank, J., Miller, J.P., Gado, M., Mckeel, M.I., et al (2005) 'Preclinical detection of Alzheimer's disease: Hippocampal shape and volume predict dementia onset in the elderly', *NeuroImage*, 25(3): 783–792.

Cummings, B.J., Head, E., Afagh, A.J., Milgram, N.W. and Cotman, C.W. (1996a) 'β-amyloid accumulation correlates with cognitive dysfunction in the aged canine', *Neurobiology of Learning and Memory*, 66(1): 11–23.

Cummings, B.J., Head, E., Ruehl, W., Milgram, N.W. and Cotman, C.W. (1996b) 'The canine as an animal model of human aging and dementia', *Neurobiology of Aging*, 17(2): 259–268.

Cummings, B.J., Satou, T., Head, E., Milgram, N.W., Cole, G.M., Savage, M.J., et al (1996c) 'Diffuse plaques contain C-terminal A beta 42 and not A beta 40: Evidence from cats and dogs', *Neurobiology of Aging*, 17(4): 653–659.

Dekosky, S.T. and Scheff, S.W. (1990) 'Synapse loss in frontal cortex biopsies in Alzheimer's disease: Correlation with cognitive severity', *Annals of Neurology: Official Journal of the American Neurological Association and the Child Neurology Society*, 27(5): 457–464.

Den Heijer, T., Geerlings, M.I., Hoebeek, F.E., Hofman, A., Koudstaal, P.J. and Breteler, M.M. (2006) 'Use of hippocampal and amygdalar volumes on magnetic resonance imaging to predict dementia in cognitively intact elderly people', *Archives of General Psychiatry*, 63(1): 57–62.

Dickerson, B.C., Stoub, T.R., Shah, R.C., Sperling, R.A., Killiany, R.J., Albert, M.S., et al (2011) 'AD signature MRI biomarker predicts AD dementia in cognitively normal adults', *Neurology*, 76(16): 1395–1402.

Dickson, D.W., Crystal, H.A., Bevona, C., Honer, W., Vincent, I. and Davies, P. (1995) 'Correlations of synaptic and pathological markers with cognition of the elderly', *Neurobiology of Aging*, 16(3): 285–298.

Fankhauser, R., Luginbühl, H. and Mcgrath, J.T. (1965) 'Cerebrovascular disease in various animal species', *Annals of the New York Academy of Sciences*, 127(1): 817–860.

Fox, M.W. (1971) *Integrative Development of Brain and Behavior in the Dog*, Chicago, IL: University of Chicago Press.

Fox, N.C., Warrington, E.K., Freeborough, P.A., Hartikainen, P., Kennedy, A.M., Stevens, J.M., et al (1996) 'Presymptomatic hippocampal atrophy in Alzheimer's disease: A longitudinal MRI study', *Brain*, 119(6): 2001–2007.

Games, D., Adams, D., Alessandrini, R., Barbour, R., Borthelette, P., Blackwell, C., et al (1995) 'Alzheimer-type neuropathology in transgenic mice overexpressing V717F β-amyloid precursor protein', *Nature*, 373(6514): 523–527.

Geula, C., Nagykery, N. and Wu, C.-K. (2002) 'Amyloid-β deposits in the cerebral cortex of the aged common marmoset (Callithrix jacchus): Incidence and chemical composition', *Acta Neuropathologica*, 103(1): 48–58.

Ghavami, S., Shojaei, S., Yeganeh, B., Ande, S.R., Jangamreddy, J.R., Mehrpour, M., et al (2014) 'Autophagy and apoptosis dysfunction in neurodegenerative disorders', *Progress in Neurobiology*, 112: 24–49.

Glass, D., Viñuela, A., Davies, M.N., Ramasamy, A., Parts, L., Knowles, D., et al (2013) 'Gene expression changes with age in skin, adipose tissue, blood and brain', *Genome Biology*, 14(7): 1–12.

Goate, A., Chartier-Harlin, M.-C., Mullan, M., Brown, J., Crawford, F., Fidani, L., et al (1991) 'Segregation of a missense mutation in the amyloid precursor protein gene with familial Alzheimer's disease', *Nature*, 349(6311): 704–706.

Goedert, M., Spillantini, M., Jakes, R., Rutherford, D. and Crowther, R. (1989) 'Multiple isoforms of human microtubule-associated protein tau: Sequences and localization in neurofibrillary tangles of Alzheimer's disease', *Neuron*, 3(4): 519–526.

Gonneaud, J., Arenaza-urquijo, E.M., Mézenge, F., Landeau, B., Gaubert, M., Bejanin, A., et al (2017) 'Increased florbetapir binding in the temporal neocortex from age 20 to 60 years', *Neurology*, 89(24): 2438–2446.

Gunn-Moore, D., Mcvee, J., Bradshaw, J.M., Pearson, G.R. and Gunn-Moore, F.J. (2006) 'Ageing changes in cat brains demonstrated by beta-amyloid and AT8-immunoreactive phosphorylated tau deposits', *Journal of Feline Medicine and Surgery*, 8(4): 234–242.

Gunn-Moore, D., Moffat, K., Christie, L.A. and Head, E. (2007) 'Cognitive dysfunction and the neurobiology of ageing in cats', *Journal of Small Animal Practice*, 48(10): 546–553.

Gunn-Moore, D., Kaidanovich-Beilin, O., Gallego Iradi, M.C., Gunn-Moore, F. and Lovestone, S. (2018) 'Alzheimer's disease in humans and other animals: A consequence of postreproductive life span and longevity rather than aging', *Alzheimers & Dementia*, 14(2): 195–204.

Hardy, J. and Allsop, D. (1991) 'Amyloid deposition as the central event in the aetiology of Alzheimer's disease', *Trends in Pharmacological Sciences*, 12(10): 383–388.

Hardy, J.A. and Higgins, G.A. (1992) 'Alzheimer's disease: The amyloid cascade hypothesis', *Science*, 256(5054): 184–186.

Harrison, J. and Buchwald, J. (1982) 'Auditory brainstem responses in the aged cat', *Neurobiology of Aging*, 3(3): 163–171.

Harrison, J. and Buchwald, J. (1983) 'Eyeblink conditioning deficits in the old cat', *Neurobiology of Aging*, 4(1): 45–51.

Hasegawa, D., Yayoshi, N., Fujita, Y. and Orima, H. (2005) 'Measurement of interthalamic adhesion thickness as a criteria for brain atrophy in dogs with and without cognitive dysfunction (dementia)', *Veterinary Radiology and Ultrasound*, 46(6): 452–457.

Head, E. and Milgram, N. (1992) 'Changes in spontaneous behavior in the dog following oral administration of L-deprenyl', *Pharmacology Biochemistry and Behavior*, 43(3): 749–757.

Head, E., Mehta, R., Hartley, J., Kameka, M., Cummings, B., Cotman, C., et al (1995) 'Spatial learning and memory as a function of age in the dog', *Behavioral Neuroscience*, 109(5): 851–858.

Head, E., Callahan, H., Cummings, B., Cotman, C., Ruehl, W., Muggenberg, B., et al (1997) 'Open field activity and human interaction as a function of age and breed in dogs', *Physiology & Behavior*, 62(5): 963–971.

Head, E., Callahan, H., Muggenburg, B., Cotman, C. and Milgram, N. (1998) 'Visual-discrimination learning ability and β-amyloid accumulation in the dog', *Neurobiology of Aging*, 19(5): 415–425.

Head, E., Mccleary, R., Hahn, F., Milgram, N. and Cotman, C. (2000) 'Region-specific age at onset of β-amyloid in dogs', *Neurobiology of Aging*, 21(1): 89–96.

Head, E., Moffat, K.S., Das, P., Sarsoza, F., Poon, W.W., Landsberg, G.M., et al (2005) 'Beta-amyloid deposition and tau phosphorylation in clinically characterized aged cats', *Neurobiology of Aging*, 26(5): 749–763.

Head, E., Pop, V., Vasilevko, V., Hill, M., Saing, T., Sarsoza, F., et al (2008) 'A two-year study with fibrillar beta-amyloid (Abeta) immunization in aged canines: Effects on cognitive function and brain Abeta', *Journal of Neuroscience*, 28(14): 3555–3566.

Hofman, A., Ott, A., Breteler, M.M., Bots, M.L., Slooter, A.J., Van Harskamp, F., et al (1997) 'Atherosclerosis, apolipoprotein E, and prevalence of dementia and Alzheimer's disease in the Rotterdam Study', *Lancet*, 349(9046): 151–154.

Houpt, K.A. and Beaver, B. (1981) 'Behavioral problems of geriatric dogs and cats', *The Veterinary Clinics of North America. Small Animal Practice*, 11(4): 643–652.

Hsiao, K., Chapman, P., Nilsen, S., Eckman, C., Harigaya, Y., Younkin, S., et al (1996) 'Correlative memory deficits, Aβ elevation, and amyloid plaques in transgenic mice', *Science*, 274(5284): 99–103.

Hwang, I.K., Yoo, K.-Y., Li, H., Choi, J.H., Kwon, Y.-G., Ahn, Y., et al (2007) 'Differences in doublecortin immunoreactivity and protein levels in the hippocampal dentate gyrus between adult and aged dogs', *Neurochemical Research*, 32(9): 1604–1609.

Insua, D., Suárez, M.-L., Santamarina, G., Sarasa, M. and Pesini, P. (2010) 'Dogs with canine counterpart of Alzheimer's disease lose noradrenergic neurons', *Neurobiology of Aging*, 31(4): 625–635.

Ishihara, T., Gondo, T., Takahashi, M., Uchino, F., Ikeda, S.-I., Allsop, D., et al (1991) 'Immunohistochemical and immunoelectron microscopical characterization of cerebrovascular and senile plaque amyloid in aged dogs' brains', *Brain Research*, 548(1–2): 196–205.

Jack, C.R. Jr., Shiung, M.M., Weigand, S.D., O'Brien, P.C., Gunter, J.L., Boeve, B.F., et al (2005) 'Brain atrophy rates predict subsequent clinical conversion in normal elderly and amnestic MCI', *Neurology*, 65(8): 1227–1231.

Jahns, H., Callanan, J.J., Maelroy, M.C. and Et, A. (2006) 'Age-related and non age-related changes in 100 surveyed horse brains', *Veterinary Pathology*, 43(5): 740–750.

Johnstone, E., Chaney, M., Norris, F., Pascual, R. and Little, S. (1991) 'Conservation of the sequence of the Alzheimer's disease amyloid peptide in dog, polar bear and five other mammals by cross-species polymerase chain reaction analysis', *Molecular Brain Research*, 10(4): 299–305.

Kametani, F. and Hasegawa, M. (2018) 'Reconsideration of amyloid hypothesis and tau hypothesis in Alzheimer's disease', *Frontiers in Neuroscience*, 12: 25.

Kaye, J.A., Swihart, T., Howieson, D., Dame, A., Moore, M.M., Karnos, T., et al (1997) 'Volume loss of the hippocampus and temporal lobe in healthy elderly persons destined to develop dementia', *Neurology*, 48(5): 1297–1304.

Kimura, N., Nakamura, S., Goto, N., Narushima, E., Hara, I., Shichiri, S., et al (2001) 'Senile plaques in an aged western lowland gorilla', *Experimental Animals*, 50(1): 77–81.

Kuroki, K., Uchida, K., Kiatipattanasakul, W., Nakamura, S., Yamaguchi, R., Nakayama, H., et al (1997) 'Immunohistochemical detection of tau proteins in various non-human animal brains', *Neuropathology*, 17(3): 174–180.

Laferla, F.M. and Green, K.N. (2012) 'Animal models of Alzheimer disease', *Cold Spring Harbor Perspectives in Medicine*, 2(11): a006320.

Landsberg, G. and Araujo, J.A. (2005) 'Behavior problems in geriatric pets', *Veterinary Clinics: Small Animal Practice*, 35(3): 675–698.

Landsberg, G.M., Hunthausen, W. and Ackerman, L. (2003) 'The effects of aging on the behavior of senior pets', in G.M. Landsberg, W. Hunthausen and L. Ackerman (eds) *Handbook of Behavior Problems of the Dog and Cat*, 2nd edn, Oxford: Saunders, pp 269–304.

Landsberg, G.M., Nichol, J. and Araujo, J.A. (2012) 'Cognitive dysfunction syndrome: A disease of canine and feline brain aging', *Veterinary Clinics: Small Animal Practice*, 42(4): 749–768.

Lee, H.-G., Perry, G., Moreira, P.I., Garrett, M.R., Liu, Q., Zhu, X., et al (2005) 'Tau phosphorylation in Alzheimer's disease: Pathogen or protector?', *Trends in Molecular Medicine*, 11(4): 164–169.

Levine, M.S., Adinolfi, A.M., Fisher, R.S., Hull, C.D., Buchwald, N.A. and McAllister, J.P. (1986) 'Quantitative morphology of medium-sized caudate spiny neurons in aged cats', *Neurobiology of Aging*, 7(4): 277–286.

Levine, M.S., Lloyd, R.L., Hull, C., Fisher, R. and Buchwald, N. (1987a) 'Neurophysiological alterations in caudate neurons in aged cats', *Brain Research*, 401(2): 213–230.

Levine, M.S., Lloyd, R.L., Fisher, R.S., Hull, C.D. and Buchwald, N.A. (1987b) 'Sensory, motor and cognitive alterations in aged cats', *Neurobiology of Aging*, 8(3): 253–263.

Levine, M.S., Lloyd, R.L., Hull, C.D., Fisher, R.S. and Buchwald, N.A. (1987c) 'Neurophysiological and morphological alterations in caudate neurons in aged cats', *Brain Research*, 401(2): 213–230.

Levine, M.S., Adinolfi, A.M., Fisher, R.S., Hull, C.D., Guthrie, D. and Buchwald, N.A. (1988) 'Ultrastructural alterations in caudate nucleus in aged cats', *Brain Research*, 440(2): 267–279.

Levy, E., Carman, M.D., Fernandez-Madrid, I.J., Power, M.D., Lieberburg, I., Van Duinen, S.G., et al (1990) 'Mutation of the Alzheimer's disease amyloid gene in hereditary cerebral hemorrhage, Dutch type', *Science*, 248(4959): 1124–1126.

Levy-Lahad, E., Wasco, W., Poorkaj, P., Romano, D.M., Oshima, J., Pettingell, W.H., et al (1995) 'Candidate gene for the chromosome 1 familial Alzheimer's disease locus', *Science*, 269(5226): 973–977.

Lewis, J., Dickson, D.W., Lin, W.-L., Chisholm, L., Corral, A., Jones, G., et al (2001) 'Enhanced neurofibrillary degeneration in transgenic mice expressing mutant tau and APP', *Science*, 293(5534): 1487–1491.

Madari, A., Farbakova, J., Katina, S., Smolek, T., Novak, P., Weissova, T., et al (2015) 'Assessment of severity and progression of canine cognitive dysfunction syndrome using the CAnine DEmentia Scale (CADES)', *Applied Animal Behaviour Science*, 171: 138–145.

Malbon, A.J., Sordo, L., Wilson, L.A., Paraschou, G., Macintyre, N., Gunn-Moore, D., et al (2022) 'Alzheimer-like pathology in the parietal cortex and hippocampus of aged donkeys: A preliminary investigation', *Neurobiology of Aging*, 113: 7–14.

Mandara, M.T. (2003) 'Meningial blood vessel calcification in the brain of the cat', *Acta Neuropathologica*, 105(3): 240–244.

Markowska, A.L., Stone, W.S., Ingram, D.K., Reynolds, J., Gold, P.E., Conti, L.H., et al (1989) 'Individual differences in aging: Behavioral and neurobiological correlates', *Neurobiology of Aging*, 10(1): 31–43.

Márquez, M., Serafin, A., Fernandez-Bellon, H., Serrat, S., Ferrer-Admetlla, A., Bertranpetit, J., et al (2008) 'Neuropathologic findings in an aged albino gorilla', *Veterinary Pathology*, 45(4): 531–537.

Martin, S.B., Smith, C.D., Collins, H.R., Schmitt, F.A. and Gold, B.T. (2011) 'Evidence that volume of anterior medial temporal lobe is reduced in seniors destined for mild cognitive impairment', *Neurobiology of Aging*, 31(7): 1099–1106.

Martínez, J., Montgomery, D.L. and Uzal, F.A. (2012) 'Vascular mineralization in the brain of horses', *Journal of Veterinary Diagnostic Investigation*, 24(3): 612–617.

Melis, J.P., Jonker, M.J., Vijg, J., Hoeijmakers, J.H., Breit, T.M. and Van Steeg, H. (2013) 'Aging on a different scale: Chronological versus pathology-related aging', *Aging (Albany NY)*, 5(10): 782–788.

Milgram, N.W., Head, E., Weiner, E. and Thomas, E. (1994) 'Cognitive functions and aging in the dog: Acquisition of nonspatial visual tasks', *Behavioral Neuroscience*, 108(1): 57–68.

Milgram, N.W., Adams, B., Callahan, H., Head, E., Mackay, B., Thirlwell, C., et al (1999) 'Landmark discrimination learning in the dog', *Learning & Memory*, 6(1): 54–61.

Milgram, N.W., Head, E., Muggenburg, B., Holowachuk, D., Murphey, H., Estrada, J., et al (2002) 'Landmark discrimination learning in the dog: Effects of age, an antioxidant fortified food, and cognitive strategy', *Neuroscience & Biobehavioral Reviews*, 26(6): 679–695.

Milgram, N.W., Landsberg, G.M., De Rivera, C. and Al, E. (2011) 'Age and cognitive dysfunction in the domestic cat', *Proceedings of the ACVB/AVSAB Symposium, St. Louis, MO*, pp 28–29.

Miller, A., Alston, R. and Corsellis, J. (1980) 'Variation with age in the volumes of grey and white matter in the cerebral hemispheres of man: Measurements with an image analyser', *Neuropathology and Applied Neurobiology*, 6(2): 119–132.

Moffat, K. and Landsberg, G. (2003) 'An investigation of the prevalence of clinical signs of cognitive dysfunction syndrome (CDS) in cats', *Journal of the American Animal Hospital Association*, 39(512): 10–5326.

Mondragón-Rodríguez, S., Perry, G., Luna-Muñoz, J., Acevedo-Aquino, M.C. and Williams, S. (2014) 'Phosphorylation of tau protein at sites Ser(396–404) is one of the earliest events in Alzheimer's disease and Down syndrome', *Neuropathology and Applied Neurobiology*, 40(2): 121–135.

Morris, J.C., Roe, C.M., Grant, E.A., Head, D., Storandt, M., Goate, A.M., et al (2009) 'Pittsburgh compound B imaging and prediction of progression from cognitive normality to symptomatic Alzheimer disease', *Archives of Neurology*, 66(12): 1469–1475.

Muir, J.L. (1997) 'Acetylcholine, aging, and Alzheimer's disease', *Pharmacology, Biochemistry, and Behavior*, 56(4): 687–696.

Nakamura, S., Tamaoka, A., Sawamura, N., Nakayama, H., Ono, F., Sakakibara, I., et al (1995) 'Carboxyl end-specific monoclonal antibodies to amyloid β protein (Aβ) subtypes (Aβ40 and Aβ42 (43)) differentiate Aβ in senile plaques and amyloid angiopathy in brains of aged cynomolgus monkeys', *Neuroscience Letters*, 201(2): 151–154.

Nakamura, S., Nakayama, H., Kiatipattanasakul, W., Uetsuka, K., Uchida, K. and Goto, N. (1996) 'Senile plaques in very aged cats', *Acta Neuropathologica*, 91(4): 437–439.

Neilson, J.C., Hart, B.L., Cliff, K.D. and Ruehl, W.W. (2001) 'Prevalence of behavioral changes associated with age-related cognitive impairment in dogs', *Journal of the American Veterinary Medical Association*, 218(11): 1787–1791.

Nelson, P.T., Greenberg, S.G. and Saper, C.B. (1994) 'Neurofibrillary tangles in the cerebral cortex of sheep', *Neuroscience Letters*, 170(1): 187–190.

Nelson, P.T., Schmitt, F.A., Lin, Y., Abner, E.L., Jicha, G.A., Patel, E., et al (2011) 'Hippocampal sclerosis in advanced age: Clinical and pathological features', *Brain*, 134(5): 1506–1518.

Noh, D., Choi, S., Choi, H., Lee, Y. and K.L. (2017) 'Evaluation of interthalamic adhesion size as an indicator of brain atrophy in dogs with and without cognitive dysfunction', *Veterinary Radiology and Ultrasound*, 58(5): 581–587.

Oikawa, N., Kimura, N. and Yanagisawa, K. (2010) 'Alzheimer-type tau pathology in advanced aged nonhuman primate brains harboring substantial amyloid deposition', *Brain Research*, 1315: 137–149.

O'Neill, D.G., Church, D.B., McGreevy, P.D., Thomson, P.C. and Brodbelt, D.C. (2015) 'Longevity and mortality of cats attending primary care veterinary practices in England', *Journal of Feline Medicine and Surgery*, 17(2): 125–133.

Pekcec, A., Baumgärtner, W., Bankstahl, J.P., Stein, V.M. and Potschka, H. (2008) 'Effect of aging on neurogenesis in the canine brain', *Aging Cell*, 7(3): 368–374.

Perl, D.P. (2010) 'Neuropathology of Alzheimer's disease', *Mount Sinai Journal of Medicine: A Journal of Translational and Personalized Medicine*, 77(1): 32–42.

Poduri, A., Gearing, M., Rebeck, G.W., Mirra, S.S., Tigges, J. and Hyman, B.T. (1994) 'Apolipoprotein E4 and beta amyloid in senile plaques and cerebral blood vessels of aged rhesus monkeys', *The American Journal of Pathology*, 144(6): 1183–1187.

Pugliese, M., Gangitano, C., Ceccariglia, S., Carrasco, J.L., Del Fà, A., Rodríguez, M.J., et al (2007) 'Canine cognitive dysfunction and the cerebellum: Acetylcholinesterase reduction, neuronal and glial changes', *Brain Research*, 1139: 85–94.

Pugliese, M., Carrasco, J.L., Gomez-Anson, B., Andrade, C., Zamora, A., Rodriguez, M.J., et al (2010) 'Magnetic resonance imaging of cerebral involutional changes in dogs as markers of aging: An innovative tool adapted from a human visual rating scale', *The Veterinary Journal*, 186(2): 166–171.

Rapp, P. (1993) 'Neuropsychological analysis of learning and memory in the aged nonhuman primate', *Neurobiology of Aging*, 14(6): 627–629.

Rapp, P.R. and Amaral, D.G. (1991) 'Recognition memory deficits in a subpopulation of aged monkeys resemble the effects of medial temporal lobe damage', *Neurobiology of Aging*, 12(5): 481–486.

Raz, N. (2004) 'The ageing brain: Structural changes and their implications for cognitive ageing', in R. Dixon, L. Backman and L. Nilsson (eds) *New Frontiers in Cognitive Aging*, Oxford: Oxford University Press.

Raz, N., Gunning, F.M., Head, D., Dupuis, J.H., Mcquain, J., Briggs, S.D., et al (1997) 'Selective aging of the human cerebral cortex observed in vivo: Differential vulnerability of the prefrontal gray matter', *Cerebral Cortex (New York, NY: 1991)*, 7(3): 268–282.

Reid, S.J., McKean, N.E., Henty, K., Portelius, E., Blennow, K., Rudiger, S.R., et al (2017) 'Alzheimer's disease markers in the aged sheep (Ovis aries)', *Neurobiology of Aging*, 58: 112–119.

Revesz, T., Holton, J.L., Lashley, T., Plant, G., Rostagno, A., Ghiso, J., et al (2002) 'Sporadic and familial cerebral amyloid angiopathies', *Brain Pathology*, 12(3): 343–357.

Revesz, T., Ghiso, J., Lashley, T., Plant, G., Rostagno, A., Frangione, B., et al (2003) 'Cerebral amyloid angiopathies: A pathologic, biochemical, and genetic view', *Journal of Neuropathology & Experimental Neurology*, 62(9): 885–898.

Ricciarelli, R. and Fedele, E. (2017) 'The amyloid cascade hypothesis in Alzheimer's disease: It's time to change our mind', *Current Neuropharmacology*, 15(6): 926–935.

Rink, C. and Khanna, S. (2011) 'Significance of brain tissue oxygenation and the arachidonic acid cascade in stroke', *Antioxidants & Redox Signaling*, 14(10): 1889–1903.

Roertgen, K.E., Parisi, J.E., Clark, H.B., Barnes, D.L., O'Brien, T.D. and Johnson, K.H. (1996) 'Aβ-associated cerebral angiopathy and senile plaques with neurofibrillary tangles and cerebral hemorrhage in an aged wolverine (Gulo gulo)', *Neurobiology of Aging*, 17(2): 243–247.

Rogaev, E., Sherrington, R., Rogaeva, E., Levesque, G., Ikeda, M., Liang, Y., et al (1995) 'Familial Alzheimer's disease in kindreds with missense mutations in a gene on chromosome 1 related to the Alzheimer's disease type 3 gene', *Nature*, 376(6543): 775–778.

Rosen, R.F., Farberg, A.S., Gearing, M., Dooyema, J.M., Long, P., Anderson, D.C., et al (2008) 'Tauopathy with paired helical filaments in an aged chimpanzee', *Journal of Comparative Neurology*, 509(3): 259–270.

Salvin, H.E., Mcgreevy, P.D., Sachdev, P.S. and Valenzuela, M.J. (2011) 'The canine cognitive dysfunction rating scale (CCDR): A data-driven and ecologically relevant assessment tool', *The Veterinary Journal*, 188(3): 331–336.

Schindowski, K., Bretteville, A., Leroy, K., Bégard, S., Brion, J.-P., Hamdane, M., et al (2006) 'Alzheimer's disease-like tau neuropathology leads to memory deficits and loss of functional synapses in a novel mutated tau transgenic mouse without any motor deficits', *The American Journal of Pathology*, 169(2): 599–616.

Schmidt, F., Boltze, J., Jäger, C., Hofmann, S., Willems, N., Seeger, J., et al (2015) 'Detection and quantification of β-amyloid, pyroglutamyl Aβ, and tau in aged canines', *Journal of Neuropathology and Experimental Neurology*, 74(9): 912–923.

Schultz, C., Dehghani, F., Hubbard, G.B., Thal, D.R., Struckhoff, G., Braak, E., et al (2000a) 'Filamentous tau pathology in nerve cells, astrocytes, and oligodendrocytes of aged baboons', *Journal of Neuropathology and Experimental Neurology*, 59(1): 39–52.

Schultz, C., Hubbard, G., Rüb, U., Braak, E. and Braak, H. (2000b) 'Age-related progression of tau pathology in brains of baboons', *Neurobiology of Aging*, 21(6): 905–912.

Selkoe, D.J. (1997) 'Alzheimer's disease: Genotypes, phenotype, and treatments', *Science*, 275(5300): 630–631.

Selkoe, D.J., Bell, D.S., Podlisny, M.B., Price, D.L. and Cork, L.C. (1987) 'Conservation of brain amyloid proteins in aged mammals and humans with Alzheimer's disease', *Science*, 235(4791): 873–877.

Serizawa, S., Chambers, J. and Une, Y. (2012) 'Beta amyloid deposition and neurofibrillary tangles spontaneously occur in the brains of captive cheetahs (Acinonyx jubatus)', *Veterinary Pathology*, 49(2): 304–312.

Serrano-Pozo, A., Frosch, M.P., Masliah, E. and Hyman, B.T. (2011a) 'Neuropathological alterations in Alzheimer disease', *Cold Spring Harbor Perspectives in Medicine*, 1(1): a006189.

Serrano-Pozo, A., Mielke, M.L., Gómez-Isla, T., Betensky, R.A., Growdon, J.H., Frosch, M.P., et al (2011b) 'Reactive glia not only associates with plaques but also parallels tangles in Alzheimer's disease', *The American Journal of Pathology*, 179(3): 1373–1384.

Šimić, G., Kostović, I., Winblad, B. and Bogdanović, N. (1997) 'Volume and number of neurons of the human hippocampal formation in normal aging and Alzheimer's disease', *Journal of Comparative Neurology*, 379(4): 482–494.

Siwak, C.T., Tapp, P.D. and Milgram, N.W. (2001) 'Effect of age and level of cognitive function on spontaneous and exploratory behaviors in the beagle dog', *Learning & Memory*, 8(6): 317–325.

Siwak-Tapp, C.T., Head, E., Muggenburg, B.A., Milgram, N.W. and Cotman, C.W. (2007) 'Neurogenesis decreases with age in the canine hippocampus and correlates with cognitive function', *Neurobiology of Learning and Memory*, 88(2): 249–259.

Siwak-Tapp, C.T., Head, E., Muggenburg, B.A., Milgram, N.W. and Cotman, C.W. (2008) 'Region specific neuron loss in the aged canine hippocampus is reduced by enrichment', *Neurobiology of Aging*, 29(1): 39–50.

Smolek, T., Madari, A., Farbakova, J., Kandrac, O., Jadhav, S., Cente, M., et al (2016) 'Tau hyperphosphorylation in synaptosomes and neuroinflammation are associated with canine cognitive impairment', *Journal of Comparative Neurology*, 524(4): 874–895.

Sordo, L. and Gunn-Moore, D. (2021) 'Cognitive dysfunction in cats: Update on neuropathological and behavioural changes plus clinical management', *Veterinary Record*, 188: e3.

Sordo, L., Martini, A.C., Houston, E.F., Head, E. and Gunn-Moore, D. (2021) 'Neuropathology of aging in cats and its similarities to human Alzheimer's Disease', *Frontiers in Aging*, 2: 684607, doi: 10.3389/fragi.2021.684607

St George-Hyslop, P.H., Tanzi, R.E., Polinsky, R.J., Haines, J.L., Nee, L., Watkins, P.C., et al (1987) 'The genetic defect causing familial Alzheimer's disease maps on chromosome 21', *Science*, 235(4791): 885–890.

Studzinski, C.M., Christie, L.-A., Araujo, J.A., Burnham, W.M., Head, E., Cotman, C.W., et al (2006) 'Visuospatial function in the beagle dog: An early marker of cognitive decline in a model of human aging and dementia', *Neurobiology of Learning and Memory*, 86(2): 197–204.

Sturchler-Pierrat, C., Abramowski, D., Duke, M., Wiederhold, K.-H., Mistl, C., Rothacher, S., et al (1997) 'Two amyloid precursor protein transgenic mouse models with Alzheimer disease-like pathology', *Proceedings of the National Academy of Sciences*, 94(24): 13287–13292.

Su, M.Y., Head, E., Brooks, W.M., Wang, Z., Muggenburg, B.A., Adam, G.E., et al (1998) 'Magnetic resonance imaging of anatomic and vascular characteristics in a canine model of human aging', *Neurobiology of Aging*, 19(5): 479–485.

Svennerholm, L., Bostrom, K. and Jungbjer, B. (1997) 'Changes in weight and compositions of major membrane components of human brain during the span of adult human life of Swedes', *Acta Neuropathologica*, 94(4): 345–352.

Tapp, P.D., Siwak, C.T., Estrada, J., Head, E., Muggenburg, B.A., Cotman, C.W., et al (2003) 'Size and reversal learning in the beagle dog as a measure of executive function and inhibitory control in aging', *Learning & Memory*, 10(1): 64–73.

Tapp, P.D., Siwak, C.T., Gao, F.Q., Chiou, J.-Y., Black, S.E., Head, E., et al (2004a) 'Frontal lobe volume, function, and β-amyloid pathology in a canine model of aging', *Journal of Neuroscience*, 24(38): 8205–8213.

Tapp, P.D., Siwak, C.T., Gao, F.Q., Chiou, J.Y., Black, S.E., Head, E., et al (2004b) 'Frontal lobe volume, function, and beta-amyloid pathology in a canine model of aging', *Journal of Neuroscience*, 24(38): 8205–8213.

Tarragon, E., Lopez, D., Estrada, C., Ana, G.C., Schenker, E., Pifferi, F., et al (2013) 'Octodon degus: A model for the cognitive impairment associated with Alzheimer's Disease', *CNS Neuroscience & Therapeutics*, 19(9): 643–648.

Tekirian, T.L., Cole, G.M., Russell, M.J., Yang, F., Weikstein, D.R., Patel, E., et al (1996) 'Carboxy terminal of β-amyloid deposits in aged human, canine, and polar bear brains', *Neurobiology of Aging*, 17(2): 249–257.

Teng, K.T.-Y., Brodbelt, D.C., Pegram, C., Church, D.B. and O'Neill, D.G. (2022) 'Life tables of annual life expectancy and mortality for companion dogs in the United Kingdom', *Scientific Reports*, 12(1): 1–11.

Terry, R.D., Masliah, E., Salmon, D.P., Butters, N., Deteresa, R., Hill, R., et al (1991) 'Physical basis of cognitive alterations in Alzheimer's disease: Synapse loss is the major correlate of cognitive impairment', *Annals of Neurology: Official Journal of the American Neurological Association and the Child Neurology Society*, 30(4): 572–580.

Thal, D.R., Rüb, U., Orantes, M. and Braak, H. (2002) 'Phases of Aβ-deposition in the human brain and its relevance for the development of AD', *Neurology*, 58(12): 1791–1800.

Uchida, K., Miyauchi, Y., Nakayama, H. and Goto, N. (1990) 'Amyloid angiopathy with cerebral hemorrhage and senile plaque in aged dogs', *Nihon Juigaku Zasshi, the Japanese Journal of Veterinary Science*, 52(3): 605–611.

Uchida, K., Nakayama, H. and Goto, N. (1991) 'Pathological studies on cerebral amyloid angiopathy, senile plaques and amyloid deposition in visceral organs in aged dogs', *Journal of Veterinary Medical Science*, 53(6): 1037–1042.

Uniprot Consortium (2023) 'UniProt: The Universal Protein Knowledgebase in 2023', *Nucleic Acids Research*, 51(D1): D523–D531.

Vacher, M.C., Durrant, C.S., Rose, J., Hall, A.J., Spires-Jones, T.L., Gunn-Moore, F., et al (2022) 'Alzheimer's disease-like neuropathology in three species of oceanic dolphin', *European Journal of Neuroscience*, 57(7): 1161–1179.

Van Oijen, M., De Jong, F.J., Witteman, J.C., Hofman, A., Koudstaal, P.J. and Breteler, M.M. (2007) 'Atherosclerosis and risk for dementia', *Annals of Neurology*, 61(5): 403–410.

Vite, C.H. and Head, E. (2014) 'Aging in the canine and feline brain', *Veterinary Clinics: Small Animal Practice*, 44(6): 1113–1129.

Vite, C.H., Insko, E.K., Schotland, H.M., Panckeri, K. and Hendricks, J.C. (1997) 'Quantification of cerebral ventricular volume in English bulldogs', *Veterinary Radiology and Ultrasound*, 38(6): 437–443.

Volloch, V., Olsen, B. and Rits, S. (2020) 'Alzheimer's Disease is driven by intraneuronally retained beta-amyloid produced in the AD-specific, βAPP-independent pathway: Current perspective and experimental models for tomorrow', *Annals of Integrative Molecular Medicine*, 2(1): 90–114.

Wegiel, J., Wisniewski, H.M., Dziewiatkowski, J., Tarnawski, M., Nowakowski, J., Dziewiatkowska, A., et al (1995) 'The origin of amyloid in cerebral vessels of aged dogs', *Brain Research*, 705(1–2): 225–234.

West, M.J. (1993) 'Regionally specific loss of neurons in the aging human hippocampus', *Neurobiology of Aging*, 14(4): 287–293.

World Health Organization (2022) 'Dementia fact sheets', *World Health Organization*, 15 March 2023. Available from: www.who.int/news-room/fact-sheets/detail/dementia [Accessed 2 April 2024].

Yanai, T., Yamoto, T., Manabe, J., Takaoka, M. and Matsunuma, N. (1987) 'X-ray microanalysis of mineralization in the thalamus of aged mice', *Nihon Juigaku Zasshi, the Japanese Journal of Veterinary Science*, 49(5): 920–922.

Yanai, T., Masegi, T., Ueda, K., Manabe, J., Teranishi, M., Takaoka, M., et al (1993) 'Spontaneous globoid mineralization in the cerebellum of rats', *Journal of Comparative Pathology*, 109(4): 447–451.

Yanai, T., Masegi, T., Kawada, M., Ishikawa, K., Fukuda, K., Yamazoe, K., et al (1994a) 'Spontaneous vascular mineralization in the brains of cows', *Journal of Comparative Pathology*, 111(2): 213–219.

Yanai, T., Masegi, T., Ueda, K., Manabe, J., Teranishi, M., Takaoka, M., et al (1994b) 'Vascular mineralization in the monkey brain', *Veterinary Pathology*, 31(5): 546–552.

Zhang, C., Hua, T., Zhu, Z. and Luo, X. (2006) 'Age related changes of structures in cerebellar cortex of cat', *Journal of Biosciences*, 31(1): 55–60.

Zhang, J.H., Sampogna, S., Morales, F.R. and Chase, M.H. (2005) 'Age-related changes in cholinergic neurons in the laterodorsal and the pedunculo-pontine tegmental nuclei of cats: a combined light and electron microscope study', *Brain Research*, 1052(1): 47–55.

4

The influence of infectious disease and inflammation on neurological deficit

Anne Crilly, Stuart Woods and Fiona L. Henriquez

Introduction

There is now a growing body of evidence which supports the notion of a critical interplay between the immune system and central nervous system (CNS), with **inflammatory** mediators produced by immune cells identified as having significant impact on neurological function. Exposure to microorganisms (for example, bacteria, viruses or parasites) drives an inflammatory response by immune cells which is subsequently used to clear the infection from the body. While inflammation occurs as a regulated response to infection, conditions such as ageing, autoimmune disease, cardiovascular disease, obesity and cancer are associated with a chronic inflammatory phenotype which is often referred to as a 'sterile' inflammation. This chapter will focus on inflammation, which can occur as a result of infection by microorganisms or as the consequence of other non-infectious disease, and the mechanisms by which it can contribute to pathology associated with neurological deficit in conditions such as Alzheimer's disease.

The immune response

The immune response is a cascade of events which have evolved to defend against infection. It starts with the interaction of innate cells that constitute the first line of immune defence (such as macrophages, dendritic cells and neutrophils) with invading bacterial, viral or parasitic **pathogens** (microbes that cause infection). Key to this interaction is the ability of these cells to recognise 'non-self' molecules present on the infecting agent but not on the host's cells. The cells of the innate response trigger an inflammatory event through the release of cytokines: chemical messengers which recruit additional innate cells to the infection site to control the spread in a non-specific manner. The adaptive immune system comes into play when antigen presenting cells of the innate immune system present foreign antigen to T and B lymphocytes. These cells express specific receptors, which upon binding to foreign antigen begin a pathogen specific cell mediated and humoral response to clear the pathogen.

Innate and adaptive immunity

The first line of defence are the physical barriers of the body such as the epithelial layer of the gut and airway, and the secretions which protect them (Peterson and Artis, 2014; Eyerich et al, 2018). These barriers are also colonised by a **microbiome** (Panwar et al, 2021) which plays a key role in human health (Ding et al, 2019) including protection from infection through priming the immune system and the production of antimicrobial metabolites to inhibit potential pathogenic organisms.

If these physical barriers are breached, pathogens are first identified by cells of the innate immune system such as neutrophils, macrophages, monocytes, dendritic cells and natural killer cells. These cells recognise pathogen associated molecular patterns (PAMPs) present on pathogens but not on the host cells and include molecules such as lipopolysaccharide, flagellin, double-stranded RNA, and unmethylated CpG-DNA (Mogensen, 2009). These PAMPS are recognised by pattern recognition receptors such as toll-like receptors and nucleotide-binding and oligomerisation domain-like receptors (Mogensen, 2009). The cells of the innate immune system act to control the infection through phagocytosis, the production of reactive oxygen species and antimicrobial peptides and proteins (McDermott, 2004) as well as cytokines and chemokines which recruit immune cells to the site of infection and drive the inflammatory response to the infection. The complement cascade is a part of the humoral **innate immunity**. These are a group of plasma proteins which can be directly activated by microbes which may result in their destruction and further drive the inflammatory cascade (Paludan et al, 2021).

The innate immune system acts non-specifically to control an infection but for complete resolution the adaptive immune system needs to be activated which provides a pathogen specific immune response (Netea et al, 2019). Innate cells known as antigen presenting cells uptake and process microbial antigen and present it to T lymphocytes in the context of MHC II (**Major Histocompatibility Complex** Class II). This triggers cellular proliferation, differentiation, effector function development and migration to the site of response. CD4+ T cells, known as T helper cells, coordinate and regulate this immune response through the production of inflammatory and anti-inflammatory cytokines. The profile of these cytokines very much depends on the CD4+ T helper phenotype (Th1/Th2/Th9/Th17/Th22/Treg) induced by the infection (Dong, 2021). The cytokines control cell recruitment, activation of CD8+ cytotoxic T cells and further activate the antimicrobial activities of innate immune cells such as macrophages and neutrophils (Nandi and Behar, 2011). Activated CD8+ cytotoxic T cells recognise microbial antigen in the context of MHC I and are capable of directly killing infected cells.

Cytokines and inflammation and impact on neuronal function

The immune response is primarily mediated through the actions of small soluble proteins known as cytokines. These molecules are secreted from a range of cell types and serve to regulate the inflammatory response, with the cascade of cytokines being a fine balance between pro-inflammatory cytokines (IL-1β, IL-6, TNFα and type 1 interferons), anti-inflammatory (IL-4, IL-10, IL-13) and regulatory (IL-35, IL-27, TGFβ) cytokines. They may act either as chemical messengers between immune cells, triggering the activation and proliferation of immune cells, and some may alter metabolic process in non-immune cells or induce apoptosis (Liu et al, 2021). Some are capable of directly modifying the behaviour of the infected host such as increased pro-inflammatory cytokines such as IL-1β, IL-6, TNFα and type 1 interferons, inducing reduced mobility and motivation (Erickson and Banks, 2011). Cytokines have also demonstrated an ability to alter memory function with reduced IL-4 associated with reduced spatial awareness (Derecki et al, 2010) and reduced IL-17 signalling being associated with impairment of short-term memory (Ribeiro et al, 2019).

L-tryptophan is an essential amino acid which plays a key role in the metabolic process which derive melatonin, indole-pyruvate and serotonin. Serotonin is a key neuronal transmitter which is thought to play key roles in sleep and mood, among other functions (Jenkins et al, 2016). Tryptophan is catabolised by IL4i1 (interleukin 4 induced 1) to indole-pyruvate, by TPH (tryptophan hydrolase) to serotonin and IDO1 (indoleamine 2,3 -dioxygenase 1) to N-formyl kynurenine. IDO expression has been demonstrated to be under the regulation of pro-inflammatory cytokines such as IFNϒ. This has the effect of depleting tryptophan levels and has been tied to the successful control of several pathogens such as *Chlamydia* sp, *Toxoplasma gondii* and *Mycobacterium tuberculosis* (Pfefferkorn, 1984; Zhang et al, 2013b; Bonner et al, 2014) which are tryptophan **auxotrophs**. However, in addition to this apparent protective role of immune-mediated depletion of tryptophan, it has been linked with the development of depression-like symptoms because of increased pro-inflammatory signals in murine models (O'Connor et al, 2009a; 2009b; 2009c).

As can be seen in Figure 4.1, immune insult triggers the recruitment of macrophages and other antigen presenting cells to the brain. This results in the activation and polarisation of CD4+ T cells which drive the activation of microglial and astrocyte cells in the brain through pro-inflammatory cytokine production, which may result in neuronal damage. The pro-inflammatory

Figure 4.1: Immune responses associated with neurodegeneration

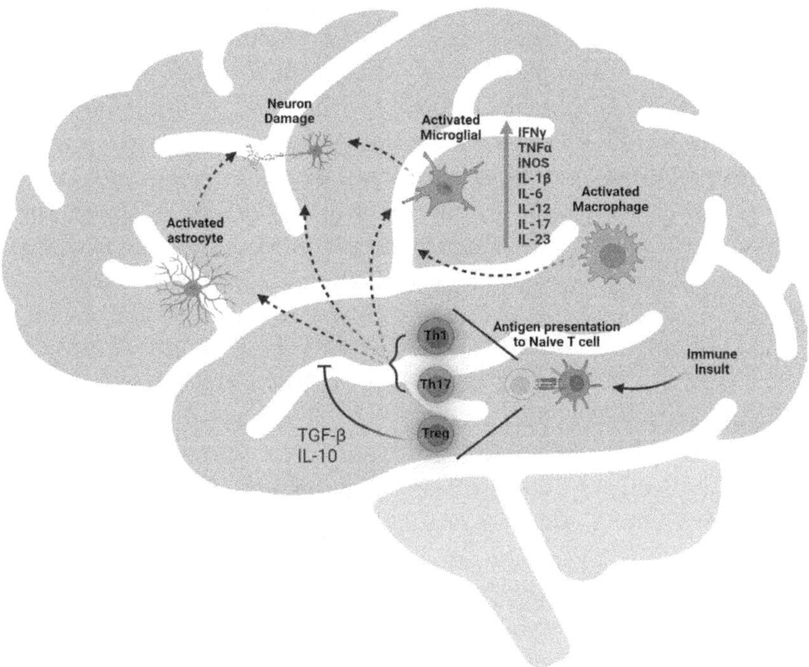

Source: Created with BioRender.com

response is countered by anti-inflammatory cytokines from a specialised population of CD4+ T cells known as T regulatory cells.

Infection-driven inflammation and neurological impairment

In the past 20 years there has been increasing interest in the possible role of infection in the brain and development of neurological conditions, including neuro-impairment. Infections that can cause chronic pro-inflammatory conditions have been associated with accelerated memory deficits and **neurodegeneration** (Fukumoto et al, 2007; Barbosa-Silva et al, 2021; Matta et al, 2021). Herein we discuss the potential impact of several infectious agents that may impact on neurological impairment.

Toxoplasma gondii

Toxoplasma gondii (*T. gondii*) is ubiquitous obligate intracellular parasite. It is estimated that up to 40 per cent of the world's population is seropositive for this infection that may go undetected or undiagnosed for the lifetime of the individual. The severity of toxoplasmosis is well characterised in the developing foetus if acquired through congenital transmission. Patients of congenital toxoplasmosis can develop cognitive and motor impairments later in life. The disease is also devastating and life-threatening in immunocompromised persons such as those with malignancies or AIDS, where toxoplasma encephalitis can destroy the CNS. Chronic infection in immunocompetent individuals was thought to be asymptomatic, but recent studies have discussed the possibility that infection in the brain can lead to neuropsychiatric disease. Specifically, toxoplasmosis has accumulated a lot of interest in recent years for its potential role to affect behaviour in its host. Immunological, epidemiological and neurological studies have shown an interaction and possible involvement in neurological conditions such as schizophrenia (Torrey and Yolken, 2007; Niebuhr et al, 2008; Arling et al, 2009; reviewed in Brown, 2006; Wang et al, 2006; Mortensen et al, 2007; Henriquez et al, 2009; Tedla et al, 2011). In rodent models *T. gondii* can cause changes in behaviour leading to reverse the aversion to the smell of cats, the parasite's definitive host, becoming the preferred odour by rodents (Berdoy et al, 2000; House et al, 2011) but speculation whether this is due to the parasite, or the immune-induced inflammation has been debated (Boillat et al, 2020). The relationship between *T. gondii* infection and Alzheimer's disease has also been scrutinised and conclusive remarks suggest that *Toxoplasma* is not involved in the aetiology as there is no significant difference in *Toxoplasma* seropositivity between patients with Alzheimer's disease and healthy volunteers (Mahami-Oskouei et al, 2016). In contrast, chronic *Toxoplasma* infection ameliorates β-amyloidosis, increasing the activity of macrophages against β amyloid plaques (Möhle et al, 2016). This has been further explored in rodent models, where the data suggests that *Toxoplasma* does not persist in the brain and therefore while pro-inflammatory molecules are produced, and there is parasite clearance, this neither positively nor negatively impacts learning and memory in ageing (McGovern et al, 2020). However, a systematic analysis of the literature by de Haan et al (2021) highlights significant association between *T. gondii* seropositivity and impaired performance of cognitive functioning (de Haan et al, 2021). In addition, a study by Yang et al (2021) reports an association between toxoplasmosis and dementia (Yang et al, 2021). From all these studies inflammation and immunological molecules are involved in neurological conditions and more research is needed to understand the mechanisms and how the immune response could be modulated to improve neuro impairment.

Helicobacter pylori

Many studies suggest a link between changes in gut microbiota and neurological disorders. Gut microbiota can communicate with the brain via neuronal, endocrine and metabolic and immunological routes, together called the microbiome–gut–brain axis. The changes in gut microbiota are typically induced through infection. *Helicobacter pylori* (*H. pylori*) is a bacterium that can colonise the stomach and establish chronic infections, demonstrating its resilience to survive in acidic conditions and evasion of the immune response. Its distribution is worldwide, and it is the named cause in peptic ulcer disease, mucosa-associated lymphoid tissue (MALT) - lymphoma, and adenocarcinoma. During infection it can change the gut microbiome, it stimulates the production of many inflammatory molecules that may have a systemic effect, thus inducing neuroinflammation and neurotoxicity (Peek et al, 2010; Alvarez-Arellano and Maldonado-Bernal, 2014). Studies also report that *H. pylori* infection can stimulate the production of free radicals and the release of neurotransmitters leading to potential dysregulation axons and neurons (Gorlé et al, 2020). Together, this presents a growing portfolio of evidence of the impact of *H. pylori* on neurological disorders. However, a longitudinal population-based study by Fani et al (2018) reported that *H. pylori* was not associated with risk of forms of dementia including Alzheimer's disease (Fani et al, 2018). Since *H. pylori* is often an asymptomatic infection, further research is needed to determine the impact of antimicrobial treatment and *H. pylori* management versus untreated asymptomatic infection.

Influenza

Influenza or 'flu' is caused by a range of influenza viruses (A, B, C, D). It is common among the human population and a variety of symptoms are associated with it ranging from mild to severe, including fever, runny nose, sore throat, muscle pain, headache, coughing and fatigue. Although, typically associated with respiratory disease it can cause diarrhoea and vomiting, particularly in children. It can progress to severe conditions, such as pneumonia, caused by the virus or by a subsequent bacterial infection leading to acute respiratory distress syndrome, meningitis, encephalitis and worsening of pre-existing health problems such as asthma and cardiovascular disease. The association with neurological impairment has also been explored establishing that the flu can impair cognitive function during infection in older patients or with recurrent infection (Bornand et al, 2016) but it does not appear to be associated with an increased risk of neurodegenerative diseases including Alzheimer's disease (Imfeld et al, 2016). In recent years attention has turned to a potential connection between dementia, Alzheimer's and the flu vaccination. There is optimism in the field as many reports conclude that vaccination may reduce the risk of the different types of dementia including Alzheimer's disease and exercise a protective role (Ali and Shaikh, 2022; Bukhbinder et al, 2022; Veronese et al, 2022). Since the principle of vaccination is to induce an immune response that memorises the target infectious agent, it is somewhat surprising that a vaccination can protect against a neurodegenerative state as pro-inflammatory products associated with the immune system are associated with neurodegeneration.

The blood brain barrier and ageing

Along with the eyes and testes, the CNS, which is the brain and spinal cord, has been long recognised as being an immunologically privileged site (Louveau et al, 2015). The brain and spinal cord are protected by the **blood brain barrier** (BBB) and the blood-cerebral spinal fluid barrier (BCB), respectively (Kadry et al, 2020). The barrier is composed of a network of microvascular structures lined with semi-permeable epithelial cells with **pericytes** (a type of fibroblast like cell intermittently found along the outside of capillaries and wrapped around the endothelial cells) identified as having a key role in maintenance of barrier function (Negi and Das, 2018). As a structure within the CNS, the BBB performs a sentinel role in that it tightly regulates the movement of molecules, nutrients and ions from the periphery into the brain. As such the barrier has a pivotal role in maintaining homeostasis, including limitation of an inflammatory response at this site. Moreover, the barrier will also protect the CNS from invading microbial pathogen, unless it becomes dysfunctional or breaks down as has been reported for bacterial infection (Peng et al, 2021) and COVID-19 (Bonetto et al, 2022). With improved imaging techniques, the dogma of 'immune privilege' for the CNS has been opened for discussion. There is now recognition that the complex interactions that exist between endothelial cells, epithelial and glial cells (includes astrocytes, microglial cells and oligodendrocytes), along with their location in the brain, means that accessibility for immune cells is possible (Engelhardt et al, 2017; Negi and Das, 2018). Moreover, under certain circumstances, the barrier system can be breached, with potentially significant consequences for CNS function. While the underlying cellular and molecular processes which lead to changes in the CNS barrier have not been fully established, ageing is known to induce changes to BBB integrity (Bowman et al, 2018; Banks et al, 2021), including increased permeability with subsequent impact on homeostasis and cognitive function. Importantly demonstrated in murine models, while ageing alters BBB integrity (Ceafalan et al, 2019), ageing and obesity together in C57BL/6 mice was found to significantly enhance BBB dysfunction along with neuroinflammation (Tucsek et al, 2014). A similar disruption has also been reported in diabetic rhesus monkeys (Xu et al, 2017) and in a murine model of Parkinson's disease (Elabi et al, 2021), with other neurodegenerative conditions such as dementia and Alzheimer's disease (Sweeney et al, 2018) also reporting BBB changes. These studies highlight the potential of certain comorbidities to significantly impact barrier integrity and CNS homeostasis. Furthermore, all of these conditions are recognised as having systemic inflammatory components which is not pathogen driven and often is referred to as a 'sterile inflammation'. The processes which drive this inflammation and the potential for this to impact neurological cognitive function will now be discussed.

Inflammaging mechanisms and neurodegenerative disease

Ageing is a complex biology which has fascinated scientists and the public for centuries. With ageing there is a significant deterioration of body systems, including vascular and cardiovascular changes which will ultimately impact blood supply to tissues, including the brain. Deterioration of the musculoskeletal system with changes to muscle (sarcopenia, which is a deficit in mass and function), bones (osteoporosis, which is a weakening of the structure, making the bone more fragile and prone to damage) and ligaments are all synonymous with the ageing process. Together these changes contribute to loss of function, with neurological impairment, frailty and disability seen as comorbidities in elderly individuals. Since the early 21st century it has been known that as we age, levels of inflammatory markers, such as immune proteins known as cytokines, including interleukin 6 (IL-6), start to elevate. This has subsequently led to the concept of **inflammaging**, a terminology first described by Claudio Franceschi in 2000 (Franceschi et al, 2000) when he observed that levels of serum inflammatory biomarkers, including cytokines, are found to increase with ageing. As inflammaging progresses, and levels of these inflammatory biomarkers increase, the risk of developing other chronic disease, such as cardiovascular disease, diabetes or dementia, with susceptibility to disability and frailty, also increases. Moreover, most of these ageing comorbidities are also known to have an inflammatory aspect. Whether this is driven specifically by ageing rather than the condition itself, is open for debate and it may be that having certain conditions with an inflammatory aspect impacts the ageing process.

Why we become more inflammatory as we get older

The mechanism by which inflammaging progresses as we age is complex and influenced by several factors, including inherited genes, environmental exposures, infection, changes in the gut microbiome and alterations to the immune system, leading to dysfunction in the response of immune cells. This has led to the identification of four key processes involved in inflammaging, which include: *cellular senescence, impairment of autophagy (a process by which cells are able to manage and clear cellular materials which are no longer needed or have become damaged), dysfunctional immune system* and *infection*. The role of infection in inflammation and neurodegeneration has been previously discussed in this chapter. The role of senescence and autophagy, along with mitophagy and meta inflammation and their impact on neurodegenerative disease will now be discussed.

Senescence is a cellular process that occurs with ageing where cell division halts in aged or damaged cells. These cells are characterised by an inflammatory **secretome**, including cytokines such as interleukin 1 (IL-1), IL-6 and tumour necrosis factor alpha (TNF α), all of which contribute to inflammaging in older individuals. Cellular senescence has been well documented in peripheral tissues during ageing and a similar process occurs with cells found in the brain, with links to Parkinson's disease (Chinta et al, 2013) and Alzheimer's disease (Guerrero et al, 2021) highlighted. Cells which are essential for brain cognitive function include endothelial cells, oligodendrocytes, microglia cells, astrocytes and neuronal cells (Baker and Petersen, 2018). All of these are susceptible to senescence with ageing and as such will have the potential to contribute to neuroinflammation and loss of cognitive function.

Autophagy is the process by which cellular debris, including used and damaged molecules, are cleared from a cell and is essential for cell function and homeostasis. Dysregulation of this process is known to occur with ageing, with changes in immune inflammatory cell profiles, such as Th17 cells which are a major source of the inflammatory cytokine, IL-17 (Bharath et al, 2020), which has been implicated in early cognitive decline in Alzheimer's (Brigas et al, 2021). Moreover, autophagy dysregulation can lead to accumulation of cellular material or debris which is also referred to as **damage associated molecular patterns (DAMPS)** which act as danger signals to the immune system (Zhang et al, 2013a). DAMPS are subsequently available to engage with innate sensing receptors found on tissue macrophages and other cells, ultimately driving the release of inflammatory mediators, including cytokines, through activation of NF–kB. Microglial cells in the brain, which are similar to tissue macrophages, can respond to DAMPS which accumulate due to impairment of autophagy, driving neuroinflammation. Disruption of autophagy has been linked to several neurodegenerative conditions, including Alzheimer's disease (Salminen et al, 2013) and Parkinson's disease (Hou et al, 2020; Badanjak et al, 2021) and will contribute to neuroinflammation through the mechanisms discussed.

In a similar process known as **mitophagy**, mitochondria that is damaged or not required is cleared from the cell. Disturbance of mitophagy, which also occurs with ageing, leads to the accumulation of damaged mitochondria and release of mitochondria DAMPS, including mitochondria DNA (mitDNA), ultimately driving inflammation and release of inflammatory mediators. The process of mitophagy is pivotal for normal cell function, including neuronal activity with several *in vivo* models used to measure this critical process (Sun et al, 2015; Fang et al, 2017). Neuronal mitophagy enhances **phagocytic** capacity of microglia cells and protects against neuronal inflammation. Like autophagy, disruption of mitophagy is known to be associated with neurodegeneration and ageing (Fivenson et al, 2017). Accumulation of damaged mitochondria is a feature of several age-related neurodegenerative conditions, including Alzheimer's disease (Kerr et al, 2017) and Parkinson's disease (Malpartida et al, 2021). Moreover, there is potential to restore cell homeostasis using mitophagy inducers such as the natural compound urolithin A which is produced in the gut by bacteria (Ryu et al, 2016) and NAD+ precursors, such as nicotinamide mononucleotide (Fang et al, 2019; Fang and Anisimov, 2023). The ability to reverse mitophagy dysfunction highlights the restorative therapeutic potential of this process. In the study by Fang et al (2019), evidence of defective mitophagy in hippocampal samples from patients with Alzheimer's disease was observed, with accumulation of damaged mitochondria in this area of the brain. In this same study, a transgenic mouse model of Alzheimer's disease was treated with mitophagy inducing agents, as was a nematode model using *C. elegans*, with significant improvement in memory observed. This study using nematodes, mice and humans demonstrates common molecular pathways linked to mitophagy dysregulation which are conserved across species and which impact significantly on cognitive function relevant to neurodegenerative disease. It is important to note that neuronal synaptic failure is the cause of memory loss and mitophagy prevents this from happening.

Therapies aimed at enhancing key cellular processes such as autophagy and mitophagy hold therapeutic promise for the future in treating neurodegenerative disease and while perhaps not a cure could be a game changer for patients living with these conditions.

Meta inflammation is a term used to describe cell metabolic changes which take place when cells are chronically exposed to an inflammatory environment. This is observed in conditions such as obesity and diabetes and has also been linked with ageing and neurodegenerative disease. Meta inflammation induces a state of chronic inflammation, leading to polarisation of macrophages with a distinctive inflammatory or M1 profile as determined by their release of mediators such as TNF α and damaging **reactive oxygen species** (ROS).

Evidence from the literature demonstrates that age-related changes in autophagy and mitophagy within the CNS are directly responsible for the accumulation of DAMPS. In turn, DAMPS will be phagocytosed by microglial cells in the brain resulting in activation and release of inflammatory molecules including IL-1 and IL-6, as well as nitric oxide and ROS, which over time will impact neuronal function (Solito and Sastre, 2012). These processes of microglial cell activation will lead to a chronic inflammatory environment within the brain which will be damaging for all cell types, potentially inducing meta inflammation and altering neuronal cell function.

The microglial cell has a pivotal role within this inflammatory cycle and therefore in neurodegenerative disease which will be further discussed.

Activation of microglial cells and neurodegenerative disease

In the brain, the microglia cells are equivalent to tissue macrophages and have a pivotal role in maintaining homeostasis within the CNS. Derived from a population of hematopoietic precursor cells during embryonic development, microglial cells are self-sustaining over a lifetime and can have both positive, as well as detrimental, effects on cognitive function. Like tissue resident macrophages in other parts of the body, microglial cells are an innate population with a critical role in host defence. While microglial cells can respond to invading brain pathogens with an inflammatory response, sustained inflammation of any kind, as can happen when there is accumulation of DAMPS within the CNS (as described previously), is detrimental for neuronal function and is a contributing factor for memory loss. While microglial cells have a key role in brain health and CNS homeostasis they are also identified as critical players in neurodegenerative conditions such as Alzheimer's disease (Lautrup et al, 2019) through various mechanisms which will be discussed.

In addition to having a role in CNS innate immunity to pathogen and breaches of the BBB, microglial cells have another important role in clearing neuronal cell debris, which they do through the process of **phagocytosis**. Neuronal mitophagy enhances the phagocytic ability of microglia cells and ultimately protects against neuronal inflammation. While these cells have an essential role in the removal of amyloid β plaques which accumulate in the Alzheimer brain (Gouras et al, 2015), they have also been implicated in the spread of Alzheimer brain pathology (Venegas et al, 2017). Amyloid β is a fragment generated from a precursor protein called amyloid. In the healthy brain, amyloid β is present in small amounts and so can dissolve in the fluid between neuronal cells. In patients with Alzheimer's disease there is an accumulation of this protein resulting in the formation of amyloid β plaques around the neurons. Consequently, these insoluble plaques have a significant impact upon neuronal function. The accumulation of amyloid β in Alzheimer's disease is also thought to be toxic to the neuronal cells. Studies in animals have suggested there is an impairment in microglial cell function and their ability to clear the plaques. This dysregulation of microglial cell phagocytosis has been directly linked to altered mitophagy (Fang et al, 2019). In the study by Fang et al (2019), microglial cells from Alzheimer's disease mice were found to have a 60 per cent reduction in mitophagy which was restored to normal through treatment with mitophagy inducing compounds.

Other structures which are present in the brain of someone with Alzheimer's disease and linked to loss of neuronal function, are neurofibrillary tangles (Bloom, 2014). These structures characteristically appear inside the neurons and are made up of a protein called tau. Both amyloid β plaques and tau protein in neurofibrillary tangles are features unique to the Alzheimer brain. Recent evidence from an *in vivo* murine model of disease has shown that amyloid β activation of microglial cells occurs upstream of neurofibrillary tangle formation and that this is dependent on activation of the intracellular protein complex known as **NLR3P inflammasome**, importantly also needed for production of the pro-inflammatory cytokine IL-1 (Ising et al, 2019). Moreover, tau protein phosphorylation has also been linked to mitophagy dysregulation (Fang et al, 2019).

Chronic systemic inflammation driven by comorbidities and neurodegenerative disease

While many neurodegenerative conditions and loss of cognitive function involve inflammation which can be explained by cellular and molecular changes linked directly with ageing, systemic inflammation which is present because of certain conditions may also have an impact. Systemic inflammation is a recognised feature of conditions such as cardiovascular disease, autoimmune conditions, diabetes, obesity and dementia. In one meta-analysis study, levels of the pro-inflammatory cytokines, IL-6 and TNF α, along with the anti-inflammatory cytokine, IL-10, were shown to be predictive of cardiovascular events in a patient population over the age of 65 years (Ramos et al, 2009). In a similar manner, autoimmune conditions, in which the immune system is overtly activated, such as rheumatoid arthritis (Matsumoto et al, 2021), see an increase in levels of systemic inflammatory biomarkers. This type of inflammatory response is often referred to as a 'sterile inflammation' as there is an absence of a specific pathogen driving the process. For many of these conditions the inflammation is chronic, and it is known that peripheral inflammation, such as that seen during autoimmune disease, has disruptive influences on the BBB (Liu et al, 2020). Indeed, autoimmune disease in which there is an excessive activation of both the innate and adaptive immune system has been linked to neuroinflammation in Parkinson's disease (De Virgilio et al, 2016), with rheumatoid arthritis linked with Alzheimer's disease and vascular dementia (Le Page et al, 2018; Figus et al, 2021). Moreover, an *in vivo* model of inflammatory bowel disease has demonstrated changes to the hippocampus with an increase in infiltration of macrophages and inflammatory cytokines (Gampierakis et al, 2021).

As well as chronic disease resulting in a systemic inflammation which has the potential to impact neurological function, other experiences such as exposure to anaesthetic and surgery in elderly, frail individuals can lead to delirium, which is a sudden and normally temporary loss of neurological function. This will now be discussed, along with the role played by systemic inflammation and overlap with dementia pathogenesis.

Delirium and dementia

Unlike dementia, in which there is a progressive and chronic loss of neurological function over a long period of time, delirium is a cognitive deficit which comes on suddenly and can last for days, weeks or even months. While delirium can occur in any age group, it is commonly seen in the frail and elderly (over the age of 65 years) post-surgery (postoperative delirium [POD]) or because of infection, such as a urinary tract infection. In those with dementia, symptoms include confusion, memory disturbance and loss of ability to concentrate. Symptoms are often more pronounced in the evenings, with disturbance of sleeping pattern also observed. With recovery from surgery and/or clearance of the infection, individuals will regain cognitive function, although for older people, the time to recover can be unpredictable and variable.

Evidence would suggest that the risk of developing delirium is increased in those individuals already diagnosed with dementia (Fong and Inouye, 2022). Moreover, the occurrence of delirium in individuals not diagnosed with dementia appears to be a risk factor for development of the condition. Whether this is because these individuals already have early, undiagnosed dementia is not clear and remains an area for further investigation. While the underlying mechanisms behind delirium are not fully understood, evidence would point to a disruption of the BBB along with an inflammatory response (either locally within the CNS or systemically) leading to a temporary deficit in neurological function. The potential mechanisms involved in the development of POD in the absence of obvious infection are now discussed.

Delirium, disruption of the blood brain barrier and inflammation

Surgery by its very nature is an invasive and highly traumatic procedure and as a result will induce a systemic inflammatory response (Corral-Velez et al, 2015; Margraf et al, 2020) which is regulated by the immune system. In addition to this, exposure to general anaesthetics can have a significant impact on the BBB, and on the interplay between the immune system and the brain (Subramaniyan and Terrando, 2019). Anaesthetic can have deleterious effects on BBB (Almutairi et al, 2016), as can pain relief, such as morphine (Liao et al, 2022). This disruption subsequently leaves the CNS vulnerable to systemic inflammatory drivers such as cytokines, which become elevated because of surgical procedure.

While POD is clinically well characterised, the underlying cellular and molecular mechanisms are still being explored. Recently there has been a growing body of evidence from both human and animal postoperative studies which implicates inflammation and neuronal injury as key drivers of POD. In humans, many of these studies have been focused on levels of biomarkers in the blood which are indicative of systemic inflammation and/or neuronal injury. These studies have measured serum levels of several small proteins, known as cytokines. Cytokines have an integral role in the function of the immune system, particularly in immune cell communication, but are also instrumental in regulating inflammatory response. In a study by Khan et al (2020), they reported that increased serum levels of the cytokines, IL-6, IL-8, IL-10 and TNF α, along with levels of C-reactive protein (CRP – an acute phase protein produced by the liver, and which is increased during inflammation) were associated with longer periods of and more severe delirium. In the same study, measurement of the alarmin (protein released in response to cell damage and distress) S100B, a biomarker of brain injury (Gonçalves et al, 2008), was associated with delirium severity (Khan et al, 2020). Importantly, biomarkers linked to inflammation (cytokines) and neuronal damage have also been reviewed in a meta-analysis (Wang et al, 2022). In this study, markers already known to have an association with Alzheimer's disease and other related dementias were evaluated in POD. It was found that there was a significant link to markers of systemic inflammation, including IL-6 and CRP, with links to other markers strongly associated with Alzheimer's neurodegeneration, such as amyloid-β and tau (Salvadó et al, 2022), or neuronal injury, including S100B (Yardan et al, 2011) and neurofilament light chain protein or NfL (Yuan and Nixon, 2021). In another meta-analysis study by Noah et al (2021), they reported that having higher levels of serum IL-6 and neoptrin (produced by activated macrophages) prior to surgery was associated with development of POD, with the type of surgery (they looked at cardiac, non-cardiac and orthopaedic surgical groups) likely to also impact (Noah et al, 2021).

S100 proteins are a family of regulatory proteins involved in Ca^{2+} binding resulting in a conformational change in protein structure and function. In the human, 25 proteins have been identified which have been implicated in an array of cellular functions, including inflammation, with links to various pathologies reported (Gonzalez et al, 2020). These proteins can act as DAMPS and have a pivotal role in regulating inflammatory response during periods of cellular stress and damage. During cell damage, S100 proteins are released into the cellular microenvironment where they can engage with innate type receptors such as toll-like receptors and RAGE (receptor for advanced glycation end products) which are expressed on immune and epithelial cells. In the CNS, RAGE expressed by murine microglial cells and neurons has been shown to be instrumental in the binding of the Alzheimer's associated protein, tau, promoting its uptake and spread, with knock down of the receptor reducing inflammation and cognitive deficit in an *in vivo* model of disease (Kim et al, 2023). Other studies in the mouse have also shown that systemic inflammation can alter CNS expression of RAGE from endothelial cells to neurons (Gasparotto et al, 2019). Moreover, engagement of RAGE with the S100 protein, S100B, drives inflammatory chemokine secretion and microglial cell migration (Bianchi et al, 2011). S100B is found in Schwann cells, a type of glial cell which has an important role in maintaining the neuron in the peripheral nervous system (Yardan et al, 2011) and is also found in astrocytes (Mori et al, 2010). Levels of S100B have been seen to be increased in frontotemporal dementia (Green et al, 1997), Alzheimer's disease (Petzold et al, 2003) and Parkinson's disease (Angelopoulou et al, 2021), linking the protein to neurological disease and highlighting its potential as a biomarker.

Functionally, S100B appears to be a double-edged sword in that it can have both protective and deleterious effects within the CNS depending on the concentrations. For example, at nanomolar (low) concentrations, S100B protein has a protective, anti-apoptotic effects on neurons, while at micromolar (high) concentrations it is toxic causing neuronal death (Sorci et al, 2010). In terms of a pathological role in Alzheimer's disease, this has been further evidenced in a murine study involving a **transgenic** mouse (Tg2576) which develops Alzheimer's disease (Hsiao et al, 1996) crossed with a transgenic mouse overexpressing human S100B (Tg-humS100B), where overexpression of S100B in Tg2576- humS100B mouse resulted in acceleration of Alzheimer's disease brain pathology (Mori et al, 2010).

Animal models have also been useful in understanding the impact of anaesthesia and surgery on neuronal injury and CNS inflammation. The hippocampus region of the brain is responsible for learning and memory. In a murine orthopaedic surgical model, it has been shown that there is significant elevation of complement components in the hippocampus region of the brain post-surgery, with changes specifically seen in microglial and astrocyte cells (Xiong et al, 2018). In the immune system, the complement pathway is a cascade of immune proteins which plays an important part in innate immunity and clearance of infection through regulation of inflammatory response. Xiong et al (2018) also found that the inflammatory cytokines, IL-6 and IL-1β, were increased in the hippocampus, with an increase in neutrophils also observed, indicating a disruption of the blood-cerebrospinal fluid barrier. Moreover, these inflammatory changes within the hippocampus could be attenuated with the administration of a specific complement antagonist, highlighting the possibility to protect and preserve CNS from surgery-induced inflammation and barrier disruption.

While POD is a recoverable neurological deficit linked to systemic inflammation and BBB disruption, understanding the complex biology involved in its development and subsequent resolution could help inform our understanding of other neurological conditions in which there is non-reversible loss of neurological function. Similarly, understanding of inflammatory processes associated with dementia and which overlap with delirium have the potential to inform approaches to either reduce or avoid POD, particularly in vulnerable patient groups, thus helping to preserve neurological reserve and functionality.

Conclusion

Going forward, a more holistic approach to better understanding the role of infection and inflammation in neurodegenerative disease is essential. More research looking at the interaction of CNS with the immune system and the impact of ageing and other comorbidities on inflammation will give new insight into the pathogenesis of conditions such as dementia and Alzheimer's disease. Through this knowledge it is hoped that new therapies will emerge which will improve management and quality of life for those individuals living with neurodegenerative conditions.

Acknowledgements

The authors would like to thank Professor Frank J. Gunn-Moore, St Andrews University, for taking the time to read through the chapter and for his insightful comments.

Glossary

adaptive immunity A specific immune response moderated and raised by the host following recognition of antigens on the pathogen.

autophagy Process by which cellular debris is cleared from a cell. It is essential for cell function and homeostasis, maintaining cell stability.

auxotrophs Organisms unable to synthesise specific compounds required for their growth.

blood brain barrier A network of microvascular structures which act as a filter for the brain, protecting against pathogen and other molecules. A similar structure is seen at the blood-cerebral spinal fluid barrier which also protects the spinal cord and maintains homeostasis.

damage associated molecular patters (DAMPS) Cell derived material or debri which is recognised by the immune system as a danger signal.

inflammaging Increased levels of pro-inflammatory mediators associated with ageing.

inflammation	Immune response to a foreign insult or physical damage, driven by specialised immune mediators.
innate immunity	The nonspecific immune response which rapidly develops against an infectious agent. Acts through recognition of evolutionary conserved features only found on pathogens.
Major Histocompatibility Complex (MHC)	A group of genes involved in the generation of specialised MHC proteins involved in presentation of antigen to T cells.
meta inflammation	Chronic low-grade inflammation which results in metabolic dysfunction.
microbiome	Commensal bacteria.
mitophagy	A cellular mechanism by which mitochondria that is damaged or not required is cleared from the cell. Like autophagy, it is essential for cell function and stability.
neurodegeneration	Degeneration of neuron function, particularly in the brain.
NLR3P inflammasome	Intracellular protein complex involved in inflammatory response to microbial infection and cell damage through the activation of caspase-1, an enzyme involved in the production of the immune proteins, interleukin 1 and 18 (IL-1 and IL-18).
pathobiome	Disease causing microbes.
pathogen	An infectious agent which can induce disease.
pericyte	Fibroblast like cell intermittently found along the outside of capillaries and wrapped around the endothelial cells.
phagocytosis	A process by which immune cells can engulf or 'eat' foreign material, such as microbes, to clear from the body. Phagocytic cells include blood monocytes and tissue macrophages, dendritic cells and neutrophils.
reactive oxygen species (ROS)	Reactive molecules which are unstable, contain oxygen and can cause damage to cells.
secretome	Everything produced or secreted by a cell.
senescence	A cellular process where arrested cell division occurs in aged or damaged cells.
transgenic	Genetically altered.

References

Ali, E. and Shaikh, A. (2022) 'Influenza vaccination and dementia risk; an unanticipated benefit?', *Ann Med Surg (Lond)*, 80: 104187.

Almutairi, M.M., Gong, C., Xu, Y.G., Chang, Y. and Shi, H. (2016) 'Factors controlling permeability of the blood-brain barrier', *Cell Mol Life Sci*, 73: 57–77.

Alvarez-Arellano, L. and Maldonado-Bernal, C. (2014) 'Helicobacter pylori and neurological diseases: Married by the laws of inflammation', *World J Gastrointest Pathophysiol*, 5: 400–404.

Angelopoulou, E., Paudel, Y.N. and Piperi, C. (2021) 'Emerging role of S100B protein implication in Parkinson's disease pathogenesis', *Cell Mol Life Sci*, 78: 1445–1453.

Arling, T.A., Yolken, R.H., Lapidus, M., Langenberg, P., Dickerson, F.B., Zimmerman, S.A., et al (2009) 'Toxoplasma gondii antibody titers and history of suicide attempts in patients with recurrent mood disorders', *J Nerv Ment Dis*, 197: 905–908.

Badanjak, K., Fixemer, S., Smajić, S., Skupin, A. and Grünewald, A. (2021) 'The contribution of microglia to neuroinflammation in Parkinson's Disease', *Int J Mol Sci*, 22: 4676.

Baker, D.J. and Petersen, R.C. (2018) 'Cellular senescence in brain aging and neurodegenerative diseases: Evidence and perspectives', *J Clin Invest*, 128: 1208–1216.

Banks, W.A., Reed, M.J., Logsdon, A.F., Rhea, E.M. and Erickson, M.A. (2021) 'Healthy aging and the blood-brain barrier', *Nat Aging*, 1: 243–254.

Barbosa-Silva, M.C., Lima, M.N., Battaglini, D., Robba, C., Pelosi, P., Rocco, P.R.M., et al (2021) 'Infectious disease-associated encephalopathies', *Crit Care*, 25: 236.

Berdoy, M., Webster, J.P. and Macdonald, D.W. (2000) 'Fatal attraction in rats infected with Toxoplasma gondii', *Proc Biol Sci*, 267: 1591–1594.

Bharath, L.P., Agrawal, M., Mccambridge, G., Nicholas, D.A., Hasturk, H., Liu, J., et al (2020) 'Metformin enhances autophagy and normalizes mitochondrial function to alleviate aging-associated inflammation', *Cell Metab*, 32: 44–55.

Bianchi, R., Kastrisianaki, E., Giambanco, I. and Donato, R. (2011) 'S100B protein stimulates microglia migration via RAGE-dependent up-regulation of chemokine expression and release', *J Biol Chem*, 286: 7214–7226.

Bloom, G.S. (2014) 'Amyloid-β and tau: The trigger and bullet in Alzheimer disease pathogenesis', *JAMA Neurol*, 71: 505–508.

Boillat, M., Hammoudi, P.M., Dogga, S.K., Pagès, S., Goubran, M., Rodriguez, I., et al (2020) 'Neuroinflammation-associated aspecific manipulation of mouse predator fear by Toxoplasma gondii', *Cell Rep*, 30: 320–334.

Bonetto, V., Pasetto, L., Lisi, I., Carbonara, M., Zangari, R., Ferrari, E., et al (2022) 'Markers of blood-brain barrier disruption increase early and persistently in COVID-19 patients with neurological manifestations', *Front Immunol*, 13: 1070379.

Bonner, C.A., Byrne, G.I. and Jensen, R.A. (2014) 'Chlamydia exploit the mammalian tryptophan-depletion defense strategy as a counter-defensive cue to trigger a survival state of persistence', *Front Cell Infect Microbiol*, 4: 17.

Bornand, D., Toovey, S., Jick, S.S. and Meier, C.R. (2016) 'The risk of new onset depression in association with influenza: A population-based observational study', *Brain Behav Immun*, 53: 131–137.

Bowman, G.L., Dayon, L., Kirkland, R., Wojcik, J., Peyratout, G., Severin, I.C., et al (2018) 'Blood-brain barrier breakdown, neuroinflammation, and cognitive decline in older adults', *Alzheimers Dement*, 14: 1640–1650.

Brigas, H.C., Ribeiro, M., Coelho, J.E., Gomes, R., Gomez-Murcia, V., Carvalho, K., et al (2021) 'IL-17 triggers the onset of cognitive and synaptic deficits in early stages of Alzheimer's disease', *Cell Rep*, 36: 109574.

Brown, A.S. (2006) 'Prenatal infection as a risk factor for schizophrenia', *Schizophr Bull*, 32: 200–202.

Bukhbinder, A.S., Ling, Y., Hasan, O., Jiang, X., Kim, Y., Phelps, K.N., et al (2022) 'Risk of Alzheimer's Disease following influenza vaccination: A claims-based cohort study using propensity score matching', *J Alzheimers Dis*, 88: 1061–1074.

Ceafalan, L.C., Fertig, T.E., Gheorghe, T.C., Hinescu, M.E., Popescu, B.O., Pahnke, J., et al (2019) 'Age-related ultrastructural changes of the basement membrane in the mouse blood-brain barrier', *J Cell Mol Med*, 23: 819–827.

Chinta, S.J., Lieu, C.A., Demaria, M., Laberge, R.M., Campisi, J. and Andersen, J.K. (2013) 'Environmental stress, ageing and glial cell senescence: A novel mechanistic link to Parkinson's disease?', *J Intern Med*, 273: 429–436.

Corral-Velez, V., Lopez-Delgado, J.C., Betancur-Zambrano, N.L., Lopez-Suñe, N., Rojas-lora, M., Torrado, H., et al (2015) 'The inflammatory response in cardiac surgery: An overview of the pathophysiology and clinical implications', *Inflamm Allergy Drug Targets*, 13: 367–370.

Degan, D., Ornello, R., Tiseo, C., Carolei, A., Sacco, S. and Pistoia, F. (2018) 'The role of inflammation in neurological disorders', *Curr Pharm Des*, 24: 1485–1501.

De Haan, L., Sutterland, A.L., Schotborgh, J.V., Schirmbeck, F. and De Haan, L. (2021) 'Association of Toxoplasma gondii seropositivity with cognitive function in healthy people: A systematic review and meta-analysis', *JAMA Psychiatry*, 78: 1103–1112.

Derecki, N.C., Cardani, A.N., Yang, C.H., Quinnies, K.M., Crihfield, A., Lynch, K.R., et al (2010) 'Regulation of learning and memory by meningeal immunity: A key role for IL-4', *J Exp Med*, 207: 1067–1080.

De Virgilio, A., Greco, A., Fabbrini, G., Inghilleri, M., Rizzo, M.I., Gallo, A., et al (2016) 'Parkinson's disease: Autoimmunity and neuroinflammation', *Autoimmun Rev*, 15: 1005–1011.

Ding, R.-X., Goh, W.-R., Wu, R.-N., Yue, X.-Q., Luo, X., Khine, W.W.T., et al (2019) 'Revisit gut microbiota and its impact on human health and disease', *Journal of Food and Drug Analysis*, 27: 623–631.

Dong, C. (2021) 'Cytokine regulation and function in T cells', *Annu Rev Immunol*, 39: 51–76.

Elabi, O., Gaceb, A., Carlsson, R., Padel, T., Soylu-Kucharz, R., Cortijo, I., et al (2021) 'Human α-synuclein overexpression in a mouse model of Parkinson's disease leads to vascular pathology, blood brain barrier leakage and pericyte activation', *Sci Rep*, 11: 1120.

Engelhardt, B., Vajkoczy, P. and Weller, R.O. (2017) 'The movers and shapers in immune privilege of the CNS', *Nat Immuno*, 18: 123–131.

Erickson, M.A. and Banks, W.A. (2011) 'Cytokine and chemokine responses in serum and brain after single and repeated injections of lipopolysaccharide: Multiplex quantification with path analysis', *Brain Behav Immun*, 25: 1637–1648.

Eyerich, S., Eyerich, K., Traidl-hoffmann, C. and Biedermann, T. (2018) 'Cutaneous barriers and skin immunity: Differentiating a connected network', *Trends in Immunology*, 39: 315–327.

Fang, E.F. and Anisimov, A. (2023) 'Turning up the NAD(+)-mitophagy axis to treat Alzheimer's disease', *Neural Regen Res*, 18: 319.

Fang, E.F., Palikaras, K., Sun, N., Fivenson, E.M., Spangler, R.D., Kerr, J.S., et al (2017) 'In vitro and in vivo detection of mitophagy in human cells, C. elegans, and mice', *J Vis Exp*, 129: 56301.

Fang, E.F., Hou, Y., Palikaras, K., Adriaanse, B.A., Kerr, J.S., Yang, B., et al (2019) 'Mitophagy inhibits amyloid-β and tau pathology and reverses cognitive deficits in models of Alzheimer's disease', *Nat Neurosci*, 22: 401–412.

Fani, L., Wolters, F.J., Ikram, M.K., Bruno, M.J., Hofman, A., Koudstaal, P.J., et al (2018) 'Helicobacter pylori and the risk of dementia: A population based study', *Alzheimers Dement*, 14: 1377–1382.

Figus, F.A., Piga, M., Azzolin, I., McConnell, R. and Iagnocco, A. (2021) 'Rheumatoid arthritis: Extra-articular manifestations and comorbidities', *Autoimmun Rev*, 20: 102776.

Fivenson, E.M., Lautrup, S., Sun, N., Scheibye-Knudsen, M., Stevnsner, T., Nilsen, H., et al (2017) 'Mitophagy in neurodegeneration and aging', *Neurochem Int*, 109: 202–209.

Fong, T.G. and Inouye, S.K. (2022) 'The inter-relationship between delirium and dementia: The importance of delirium prevention', *Nat Rev Neurol*, 18: 579–596.

Franceschi, C., Bonafè, M., Valensin, S., Olivieri, F., De Luca, M., Ottaviani, E., et al (2000) 'Inflamm-aging: An evolutionary perspective on immunosenescence', *Ann N Y Acad Sci*, 908: 244–254.

Fukumoto, Y., Okumura, A., Hayakawa, F., Suzuki, M., Kato, T., Watanabe, K., et al (2007) 'Serum levels of cytokines and EEG findings in children with influenza associated with mild neurological complications', *Brain Dev*, 29: 425–430.

Gampierakis, I.A., Koutmani, Y., Semitekolou, M., Morianos, I., Polissidis, A., Katsouda, A., et al (2021) 'Hippocampal neural stem cells and microglia response to experimental inflammatory bowel disease (IBD)', *Mol Psychiatry*, 26: 1248–1263.

Gasparotto, J., Ribeiro, C.T., Da Rosa-Silva, H.T., Bortolin, R.C., Rabelo, T.K., Peixoto, D.O., et al (2019) 'Systemic inflammation changes the site of RAGE expression from endothelial cells to neurons in different brain areas', *Mol Neurobiol*, 56: 3079–3089.

Gonçalves, C.A., Leite, M.C. and Nardin, P. (2008) 'Biological and methodological features of the measurement of S100B, a putative marker of brain injury', *Clin Biochem*, 41: 755–763.

Gonzalez, L.L., Garrie, K. and Turner, M.D. (2020) 'Role of S100 proteins in health and disease', *Biochim Biophys Acta Mol Cell Res*, 1867: 118677.

Gorlé, N., Bauwens, E., Haesebrouck, F., Smet, A. and Vandenbroucke, R.E. (2020) 'Helicobacter and the potential role in neurological disorders: There is more than helicobacter pylori', *Front Immunol*, 11: 584165.

Gouras, G.K., Olsson, T.T. and Hansson, O. (2015) 'β-Amyloid peptides and amyloid plaques in Alzheimer's disease', *Neurotherapeutics*, 12: 3–11.

Green, A.J., Harvey, R.J., Thompson, E.J. and Rossor, M.N. (1997) 'Increased S100beta in the cerebrospinal fluid of patients with frontotemporal dementia', *Neurosci Lett*, 235: 5–8.

Guerrero, A., De Strooper, B. and Arancibia-Cárcamo, I.L. (2021) 'Cellular senescence at the crossroads of inflammation and Alzheimer's disease', *Trends Neurosci*, 44: 714–727.

Henriquez, S.A., Brett, R., Alexander, J., Pratt, J. and Roberts, C.W. (2009) 'Neuropsychiatric disease and Toxoplasma gondii infection', *Neuroimmunomodulation*, 16: 122–133.

Hou, X., Watzlawik, J.O., Fiesel, F.C. and Springer, W. (2020) 'Autophagy in Parkinson's Disease', *J Mol Biol*, 432: 2651–2672.

House, P.K., Vyas, A. and Sapolsky, R. (2011) 'Predator cat odors activate sexual arousal pathways in brains of Toxoplasma gondii infected rats', *PLoS One*, 6: e23277.

Hsiao, K., Chapman, P., Nilsen, S., Eckman, C., Harigaya, Y., Younkin, S., et al (1996) 'Correlative memory deficits, Abeta elevation, and amyloid plaques in transgenic mice', *Science*, 274: 99–102.

Imfeld, P., Toovey, S., Jick, S.S. and Meier, C.R. (2016) 'Influenza infections and risk of Alzheimer's disease', *Brain Behav Immun*, 57: 187–192.

Ising, C., Venegas, C., Zhang, S., Scheiblich, H., Schmidt, S.V., Vieira-Saecker, A., et al (2019) 'NLRP3 inflammasome activation drives tau pathology', *Nature*, 575: 669–673.

Jenkins, T.A., Nguyen, J.C., Polglaze, K.E. and Bertrand, P.P. (2016) 'Influence of tryptophan and serotonin on mood and cognition with a possible role of the gut-brain axis', *Nutrients*, 8: 56.

Kadry, H., Noorani, B. and Cucullo, L. (2020) 'A blood-brain barrier overview on structure, function, impairment, and biomarkers of integrity', *Fluids Barriers CNS*, 17: 69.

Kerr, J.S., Adriaanse, B.A., Greig, N.H., Mattson, M.P., Cader, M.Z., Bohr, V.A., et al (2017) 'Mitophagy and Alzheimer's disease: Cellular and molecular mechanisms', *Trends Neurosci*, 40: 151–166.

Khan, B.A., Perkins, A.J., Prasad, N.K., Shekhar, A., Campbell, N.L., Gao, S., et al (2020) 'Biomarkers of delirium duration and delirium severity in the ICU', *Crit Care Med*, 48: 353–361.

Kim, Y., Park, H., Kim, Y., Kim, S.H., Lee, J.H., Yang, H., et al (2023) 'Pathogenic role of RAGE in tau transmission and memory deficits', *Biol Psychiatry*, 93: 829–841.

Lautrup, S., Lou, G., Aman, Y., Nilsen, H., Tao, J. and Fang, E.F. (2019) 'Microglial mitophagy mitigates neuroinflammation in Alzheimer's disease', *Neurochem Int*, 129: 104469.

Le Page, A., Dupuis, G., Frost, E.H., Larbi, A., Pawelec, G., Witkowski, J.M., et al (2018) 'Role of the peripheral innate immune system in the development of Alzheimer's disease', *Exp Gerontol*, 107: 59–66.

Liao, K., Niu, F., Hu, G. and Buch, S. (2022) 'Morphine-mediated release of astrocyte-derived extracellular vesicle miR-23a induces loss of pericyte coverage at the blood-brain barrier: Implications for neuroinflammation', *Front Cell Dev Biol*, 10: 984375.

Liu, C., Chu, D., Kalantar-Zadeh, K., George, J., Young, H.A. and Liu, G. (2021) 'Cytokines: From clinical significance to quantification', *Advanced Science*, 8: e2004433.

Liu, Y., Zhang, S., Li, X., Liu, E., Wang, X., Zhou, Q., et al (2020) 'Peripheral inflammation promotes brain tau transmission via disrupting blood-brain barrier', *Biosci Rep*, 40: BSR20193629.

Louveau, A., Harris, T.H. and Kipnis, J. (2015) 'Revisiting the mechanisms of CNS immune privilege', *Trends Immunol*, 36: 569–577.

Mahami-Oskouei, M., Hamidi, F., Talebi, M., Farhoudi, M., Taheraghdam, A.A., Kazemi, T., et al (2016) 'Toxoplasmosis and Alzheimer: Can Toxoplasma gondii really be introduced as a risk factor in etiology of Alzheimer?', *Parasitol Res*, 115: 3169–3174.

Malpartida, A.B., Williamson, M., Narendra, D.P., Wade-Martins, R. and Ryan, B.J. (2021) 'Mitochondrial dysfunction and mitophagy in Parkinson's disease: From mechanism to therapy', *Trends Biochem Sci*, 46: 329–343.

Margraf, A., Ludwig, N., Zarbock, A. and Rossaint, J. (2020) 'Systemic inflammatory response syndrome after surgery: Mechanisms and protection', *Anesth Analg*, 131: 1693–1707.

Matsumoto, H., Fujita, Y., Asano, T., Matsuoka, N., Temmoku, J., Sato, S., et al (2021) 'Association between inflammatory cytokines and immune-checkpoint molecule in rheumatoid arthritis', *PLoS One*, 16: e0260254.

Matta, S.K., Rinkenberger, N., Dunay, I.R. and Sibley, L.D. (2021) 'Toxoplasma gondii infection and its implications within the central nervous system', *Nat Rev Microbiol*, 19: 467–480.

McDermott, A.M. (2004) 'Defensins and other antimicrobial peptides at the ocular surface', *The Ocular Surface*, 2: 229–247.

McGovern, K.E., Cabral, C.M., Morrison, H.W. and Koshy, A.A. (2020) 'Aging with Toxoplasma gondii results in pathogen clearance, resolution of inflammation, and minimal consequences to learning and memory', *Sci Rep*, 10: 7979.

Mogensen, T.H. (2009) 'Pathogen recognition and inflammatory signaling in innate immune defenses', *Clin Microbiol Rev*, 22: 240–273.

Möhle, L., Israel, N., Paarmann, K., Krohn, M., Pietkiewicz, S., Müller, A., et al (2016) 'Chronic Toxoplasma gondii infection enhances β-amyloid phagocytosis and clearance by recruited monocytes', *Acta Neuropathol Commun*, 4: 25.

Mori, T., Koyama, N., Arendash, G.W., Horikoshi-Sakuraba, Y., Tan, J. and Town, T. (2010) 'Overexpression of human S100B exacerbates cerebral amyloidosis and gliosis in the Tg2576 mouse model of Alzheimer's disease', *Glia*, 58: 300–314.

Mortensen, P.B., Nørgaard-Pedersen, B., Waltoft, B.L., Sørensen, T.L., Hougaard, D. and Yolken, R.H. (2007) 'Early infections of Toxoplasma gondii and the later development of schizophrenia', *Schizophr Bull*, 33: 741–744.

Nandi, B. and Behar, S.M. (2011) 'Regulation of neutrophils by interferon-γ limits lung inflammation during tuberculosis infection', *J Exp Med*, 208: 2251–2262.

Negi, N. and Das, B.K. (2018) 'CNS: Not an immunoprivilaged site anymore but a virtual secondary lymphoid organ', *Int Rev Immunol*, 37: 57–68.

Netea, M.G., Schlitzer, A., Placek, K., Joosten, L.A.B. and Schultze, J.L. (2019) 'Innate and adaptive immune memory: An evolutionary continuum in the host's response to pathogens', *Cell Host & Microbe*, 25: 13–26.

Niebuhr, D.W., Millikan, A.M., Cowan, D.N., Yolken, R., Li, Y. and Weber, N.S. (2008) 'Selected infectious agents and risk of schizophrenia among U.S. military personnel', *Am J Psychiatry*, 165: 99–106.

Noah, A.M., Almghairbi, D., Evley, R. and Moppett, I.K. (2021) 'Preoperative inflammatory mediators and postoperative delirium: Systematic review and meta-analysis', *Br J Anaesth*, 127: 424–434.

O'Connor, J.C., André, C., Wang, Y., Lawson, M.A., Szegedi, S.S., Lestage, J., et al (2009a) 'Interferon-gamma and tumor necrosis factor-alpha mediate the upregulation of indoleamine 2,3-dioxygenase and the induction of depressive-like behavior in mice in response to bacillus Calmette-Guerin', *J Neurosci*, 29: 4200–4209.

O'Connor, J.C., Lawson, M.A., André, C., Briley, E.M., Szegedi, S.S., Lestage, J., et al (2009b) 'Induction of IDO by bacille Calmette-Guérin is responsible for development of murine depressive-like behavior', *J Immunol*, 182: 3202–3212.

O'Connor, J.C., Lawson, M.A., André, C., Moreau, M., Lestage, J., Castanon, N., et al (2009c) 'Lipopolysaccharide-induced depressive-like behavior is mediated by indoleamine 2,3-dioxygenase activation in mice', *Mol Psychiatry*, 14: 511–522.

Paludan, S.R., Pradeu, T., Masters, S.L. and Mogensen, T.H. (2021) 'Constitutive immune mechanisms: Mediators of host defence and immune regulation', *Nature Reviews Immunology*, 21: 137–150.

Panwar, R.B., Sequeira, R.P. and Clarke, T.B. (2021) 'Microbiota-mediated protection against antibiotic-resistant pathogens', *Genes & Immunity*, 22: 255–267.

Peek, R.M., Jr., Fiske, C. and Wilson, K.T. (2010) 'Role of innate immunity in Helicobacter pylori-induced gastric malignancy', *Physiol Rev*, 90: 831–858.

Peng, X., Luo, Z., He, S., Zhang, L. and Li, Y. (2021) 'Blood-brain barrier disruption by lipopolysaccharide and sepsis-associated encephalopathy', *Front Cell Infect Microbiol*, 11: 768108.

Peterson, L.W. and Artis, D. (2014) 'Intestinal epithelial cells: Regulators of barrier function and immune homeostasis', *Nat Rev Immunol*, 14: 141–153.

Petzold, A., Jenkins, R., Watt, H.C., Green, A.J., Thompson, E.J., Keir, G., et al (2003) 'Cerebrospinal fluid S100B correlates with brain atrophy in Alzheimer's disease', *Neurosci Lett*, 336: 167–170.

Pfefferkorn, E.R. (1984) 'Interferon gamma blocks the growth of Toxoplasma gondii in human fibroblasts by inducing the host cells to degrade tryptophan', *Proc Natl Acad Sci USA*, 81: 908–912.

Ramos, A.M., Pellanda, L.C., Gus, I. and Portal, V.L. (2009) 'Inflammatory markers of cardiovascular disease in the elderly', *Arq Bras Cardiol*, 92: 221–228/227–234. English/Spanish.

Ribeiro, M., Brigas, H.C., Temido-Ferreira, M., Pousinha, P.A., Regen, T., Santa, C., et al (2019) 'Meningeal γδ T cell-derived IL-17 controls synaptic plasticity and short-term memory', *Sci Immunol*, 4: eaay5199.

Ryu, D., Mouchiroud, L., Andreux, P.A., Katsyuba, E., Moullan, N., Nicolet-dit-Félix, A., et al (2016) 'Urolithin A induces mitophagy and prolongs lifespan in C. elegans and increases muscle function in rodents', *Nat Med*, 22: 879–888.

Salminen, A., Kaarniranta, K., Kauppinen, A., Ojala, J., Haapasalo, A., Soininen, H., et al (2013) 'Impaired autophagy and APP processing in Alzheimer's disease: The potential role of Beclin 1 interactome', *Prog Neurobiol*, 106–107: 33–54.

Salvadó, G., Shekari, M., Falcon, C., Operto, G., Milà-Alomà, M., Sánchez-Benavides, G., et al (2022) 'Brain alterations in the early Alzheimer's continuum with amyloid-β, tau, glial and neurodegeneration CSF markers', *Brain Commun*, 4: fcac134.

Solito, E. and Sastre, M. (2012) 'Microglia function in Alzheimer's disease', *Front Pharmacol*, 3: 14.

Sorci, G., Bianchi, R., Riuzzi, F., Tubaro, C., Arcuri, C., Giambanco, I., et al (2010) 'S100B protein, a damage-associated molecular pattern protein in the brain and heart, and beyond', *Cardiovasc Psychiatry Neurol*, 2010: 656481.

Subramaniyan, S. and Terrando, N. (2019) 'Neuroinflammation and perioperative neurocognitive disorders', *Anesth Analg*, 128: 781–788.

Sun, N., Yun, J., Liu, J., Malide, D., Liu, C., Rovira, I., et al (2015) 'Measuring in vivo mitophagy', *Mol Cell*, 60: 685–696.

Sweeney, M.D., Sagare, A.P. and Zlokovic, B.V. (2018) 'Blood-brain barrier breakdown in Alzheimer disease and other neurodegenerative disorders', *Nat Rev Neurol*, 14: 133–150.

Tedla, Y., Shibre, T., Ali, O., Tadele, G., Woldeamanuel, Y., Asrat, D., et al (2011) 'Serum antibodies to Toxoplasma gondii and Herpesvidae family viruses in individuals with schizophrenia and bipolar disorder: A case-control study', *Ethiop Med J*, 49: 211–220.

Torrey, E.F. and Yolken, R.H. (2007) 'Schizophrenia and toxoplasmosis', *Schizophr Bull*, 33: 727–728.

Tucsek, Z., Toth, P., Sosnowska, D., Gautam, T., Mitschelen, M., Koller, A., et al (2014) 'Obesity in aging exacerbates blood-brain barrier disruption, neuroinflammation, and oxidative stress in the mouse hippocampus: Effects on expression of genes involved in beta-amyloid generation and Alzheimer's disease', *J Gerontol A Biol Sci Med Sci*, 69: 1212–1226.

Venegas, C., Kumar, S., Franklin, B.S., Dierkes, T., Brinkschulte, R., Tejera, D., et al (2017) 'Microglia-derived ASC specks cross-seed amyloid-β in Alzheimer's disease', *Nature*, 552: 355–361.

Veronese, N., Demurtas, J., Smith, L., Michel, J.P., Barbagallo, M., Bolzetta, F., et al (2022) 'Influenza vaccination reduces dementia risk: A systematic review and meta-analysis', *Ageing Res Rev*, 73: 101534.

Wang, H.L., Wang, G.H., Li, Q.Y., Shu, C., Jiang, M.S. and Guo, Y. (2006) 'Prevalence of Toxoplasma infection in first-episode schizophrenia and comparison between Toxoplasma-seropositive and Toxoplasma-seronegative schizophrenia', *Acta Psychiatr Scand*, 114: 40–48.

Wang, S., Greene, R., Song, Y., Chan, C., Lindroth, H., Khan, S., et al (2022) 'Postoperative delirium and its relationship with biomarkers for dementia: A meta-analysis', *Int Psychogeriatr*, 1–14.

Xiong, C., Liu, J., Lin, D., Zhang, J., Terrando, N. and Wu, A. (2018) 'Complement activation contributes to perioperative neurocognitive disorders in mice', *J Neuroinflammation*, 15: 254.

Xu, Z., Zeng, W., Sun, J., Chen, W., Zhang, R., Yang, Z., et al (2017) 'The quantification of blood-brain barrier disruption using dynamic contrast-enhanced magnetic resonance imaging in aging rhesus monkeys with spontaneous type 2 diabetes mellitus', *Neuroimage*, 158: 480–487.

Yang, H.Y., Chien, W.C., Chung, C.H., Su, R.Y., Lai, C.Y., Yang, C.C., et al (2021) 'Risk of dementia in patients with toxoplasmosis: A nationwide, population-based cohort study in Taiwan', *Parasit Vectors*, 14: 435.

Yardan, T., Erenler, A.K., Baydin, A., Aydin, K. and Cokluk, C. (2011) 'Usefulness of S100B protein in neurological disorders', *J Pak Med Assoc*, 61: 276–281.

Yuan, A. and Nixon, R.A. (2021) 'Neurofilament proteins as biomarkers to monitor neurological diseases and the efficacy of therapies', *Front Neurosci*, 15: 689938.

Zhang, Q., Kang, R., Zeh, H.J., 3rd, Lotze, M.T. and Tang, D. (2013a) 'DAMPs and autophagy: Cellular adaptation to injury and unscheduled cell death', *Autophagy*, 9: 451–458.

Zhang, Y.J., Reddy, M.C., Loerger, T.R., Rothchild, A.C., Dartois, V., Schuster, B.M., et al (2013b) 'Tryptophan biosynthesis protects mycobacteria from CD4 T-cell-mediated killing', *Cell*, 155: 1296–1308.

5

Love, loss and animals: a posthumanist account of dementia in multi-species kinship

Elizabeth Peel, Damien W. Riggs and Nik Taylor

Introduction

It can be argued that all love is partial. We come to know those we love through our own lens, which filters our perceptions and feelings. But what happens when additional filters are applied, and how does that further render partial our relationships with those we love? What happens when we speak a different language to those we love, when species differences are involved, or cognitive decline? With regard to the latter, canine dementia is manifest through behavioural changes in older dogs such as disorientation, changes in activity and different interactions with those around them, altered sleeping patterns, and house-soiling (Landsberg et al, 2012). In this chapter we explore our relationships with three dogs we have loved: for Elizabeth, Bramble; for Damien, Willy; and for Nik, Squirt (Gillespie, 2022). While, as we discuss in this chapter, each of these relationships is distinct, what unites them is our human experience of living with a canine loved one who has dementia and, further, a loved one who others might not recognise as worthy of love and/or might undervalue the love we have for them. What also connects us as authors, as we explicate in what follows, is a commitment to finding ways to witness the voices of the animals we have loved. In this sense we offer a posthumanist account of our experiences of living with a dog with dementia. As Wolfe articulates, posthumanism:[1]

> [E]nables us to describe the human and its characteristic modes of communication, interaction, meaning, social significations, and affective investments with *greater* specificity once we have removed meaning from the ontologically closed domain of consciousness, reason, reflection, and so on. … But it also insists that we attend to the specificity of the human – its ways of being in the world, its ways of knowing, observing, and describing – by (paradoxically for humanism) acknowledging that it is fundamentally a prosthetic creative that has

> coevolved with various forms of technicity and materiality, forms that are radically 'not-human' and yet have nevertheless made the human what it is. (Wolfe, 2010: xxv, original emphasis)

Informing this chapter are a conceptual framework for understanding kinship and a heuristic for undertaking political and intellectual work, both developed in our previous work. The conceptual framework is that of critical kinship studies. As we have argued (Riggs and Peel, 2016), critical kinship studies offers a lens through which to consider human–human relationships as always already being formed in concert with human–animal relationships. Building on foundational texts on kinship (for example, Strathern, 1992a; 1992b), critical kinship studies is posthumanist in that it 'aims to identify how "the human" in humanism is constituted' (Riggs and Peel, 2016: 36). As we have previously discussed, posthumanism theoretically underpinning critical kinship studies allows examination of:

> the construction of human kinship practices, to examine who such practices exclude (both some humans and all non-human species), and to identify the ways in which such practices are naturalized. Given as human authors we are unable to problematize human kinship practices from a place outside our species, a posthumanist framework enables us to think about how claims about human kinship are made, and through which relationships (including inter-species relationships) they are made. (Riggs and Peel, 2016: 14)

Whether due to a presumed set of human/animal and culture/nature binaries that serve to prop up anthropocentrism, or because of the genuine bonds that many humans share with animals and vice versa, human kinship, we have argued, can never be seen as separate from the lives and kinship of animals (Haraway, 2003). In other words:

> [A] core component of critical kinship studies is to render visible the human in kinship studies, not simply by adding in non-human animals to our account of kinship, nor by claiming to know what kinship means for non-human animals. Rather, we suggest, critical kinship studies seeks to examine how technologies of human kinship are part and parcel of the construction of humanness (which is positioned in opposition to those who are not considered human), and thus to be 'critical' when we study kinship is to interrogate the anthropocentrism that is at the core of humanist accounts of kinship. (Riggs and Peel, 2016: 11)

In terms of the heuristic, and building on the critical kinship studies framework, we have developed the term 'queer menagerie' (Riggs et al,

2021) to refer to a political, experiential and methodological approach to understanding the intersections of human and animal lives. In terms of the present chapter, the concept of a queer menagerie is important as it allows for a consideration of what is 'displayed' when we as humans write about dementia as experienced by the animals we have loved. As we have suggested previously:

> in terms of epistemology – and different to (for example) bricolage – a queer menagerie provides a theoretical framework that does more than bring together differing standpoints for the purpose of display, but rather does so in a way that highlights the operations of power that it seeks to examine. This, then, is an inherently political epistemology. It is one that acknowledges the primacy accorded to human voices within a queer menagerie, but still seeks to find ways to focus on animal voices. (Riggs et al, 2021: 2)

Bringing together critical kinship studies and the heuristic of a queer menagerie, as we do in this chapter, serves our aim of bringing into conversation our own experiences of love and loss across species lines.[2] At the same time, both critical kinship studies and queer menagerie, we hope, offer ways of thinking about the voices of Bramble, Willy and Squirt. Certainly, we do not claim to know their thoughts, or to be able to ventriloquise their voices, however we do aim to at least make them *present* in this chapter. We understand that any methodological or heuristic devices aimed at including other animals can only ever be partial, and quite possibly anthropocentric (Hamilton and Taylor, 2017; Sutton, 2020). Yet it is important to attempt to trace where we have seen their agency, if not their voices, in action in our relationships with them. Doing this requires a form of academic writing that itself constitutes a queer menagerie: one that disrupts both standard academic writing and taken-for-granted human–animal binaries that rest upon assumptions of human exceptionalism. In effect, the question 'can we write to create further space for the multiple nonhumans around us' (Huopalainen, 2022: 960) underpins this chapter as we write in multiple voices, signalling at different turns where each of us takes the lead. We also use photographs to give depth to our accounts of Bramble, Willy and Squirt.[3] In many ways, then, a queer menagerie, as represented here, entails spanning the bridge between cross-species kin, while at the same time recognising the gaps.

In consolidating our thoughts and recollections, each chapter section provides a brief engagement with academic literature on human–animal kinship, animals and dementia, and humans and the loss of an animal companion. We then offer our own experiences and stories. While to a certain degree these sections are normatively ordered, following a trajectory from our initial relationships with Bramble, Willy and Squirt, through to their manifestations of dementia, our aim is to explore the messiness of human–animal relationships, including those involving dementia.[4] As a result, this focus on messiness befits a queer menagerie focused on displaying particular aspects of our connections with our dogs for the purpose of developing the limited academic writing on living with animals experiencing dementia, and specifically doing so by keeping animals at the centre.

Kinship, reproduction and normativities

Writing in a form that she terms 'feminist dog-writing', McHugh (2012) argues that 'queer writing' on animal companionship has constituted a form of resistance to normative assumptions about human reproduction. Specifically, she argues that in the face of pronatalist assumptions,[5] in addition to historical (and in some contexts ongoing) prohibitions against non-heterosexual people having children, many such people have chosen to form close loving kinship bonds with animals. This is evident in early lesbian texts on cat companions (Reti and Sien, 1991), for example, and in our own work we have explored the unique meanings that animals can bring to the lives of people marginalised because of gender and/or sexuality (Ellis et al, 2020; Riggs et al, 2021). Multi-species kinship, in these accounts, not only refuses pronatalist imperatives, but also resists the idea that kinship proper is only constituted by human–human relationships.[6]

At the same time, however, 'queer writing' on human–animal kinship very much engages in a form of reproduction: it both sets up new norms (and potentially homonorms) that come to constitute a form of idealised human life, as much as it serves to reproduce values and practices within queer communities.

Damien: All of my human children have come into my family via foster care. As a gay man, having human children over the past 20 years has often occurred in the face of a lack of understanding from other men that children could be a desirable part of adult life for a gay man. This is understandable, given historical prohibitions on gay men having children, and due to subsequent assumptions within gay men's communities that being gay meant freedom from a reproductive imperative. My relationship to my children – a relationship not based on genetics – has often been a further point of contention, skewing whether or not other people view my family as intelligible.

Willy joined my family when my first child was six years old. It seemed that he would benefit from a companion, and at the time I was not ready to parent another human child, so a dog it was. Willy came from an animal shelter and was given the name 'Willy (Wonka)' because one of his back legs didn't seem to work properly. Yet at least one of my heterosexual female friends assumed that we named him Willy in reference to what she presumed to be a gay man's hyperfocus on genitalia. This same friend was one who struggled to see my children as my children though was quick to assert that children who were later conceived by a lesbian couple for whom I donated gametes were 'my children'. Suffice it to say we are no longer friends. Her response to Willy and to my children speaks to a broader issue of how queer kinship is interpreted and framed by other people against existing stereotypes and assumptions about what constitutes kinship proper.

Elizabeth: Bramble was very much our 'first child',[7] as a lesbian who aspired to a human child a rescue puppy was a logistically more achievable precursor. We collected Bramble, a Border Collie/terrier crossbreed, age seven weeks with no sniff off a mother and riddled with worms. He altered our past queer kinship in displacing both our cats, sadly, and was both utterly adorable and utterly demanding, and destructive. We were sufficiently concerned about the impact on our family of having a human baby that we consulted a dog behaviourist during my pregnancy. Our clever Bramble was soon wise to this 'alpha' male's tricks. In the presence of the behaviourist there was no nuisance barking and attacking of the vacuum cleaner, hairdryer or lawnmower, just impeccable behaviour as we walked around with an empty pushchair, acclimatising.

When our 'homonormative' family of two women and a dog was changed by our baby's arrival, it transpired our concerns were fundamentally misplaced.[8] Bramble sniffed the new pack member and seemed instantly content with the new arrangement (Figure 5.1). Bramble was gentle with the human pup, tolerantly assisting them in learning to stand as handfuls of fur were grasped, or eyes or nose were clumsily prodded. The only child and the solo dog formed a symbiotic partnership through mutual interests in play (fetch, tug-of-war and bubble catching), which deepened over many years.

Nik: Squirt joined my family after turning up at a friend's house for several nights in a row, in winter, freezing and hungry. When attempts to contact the owner led to abuse and a parting shot to 'keep her', my friend contacted me and we (two humans and another dog, Bess) went to meet Squirt. She immediately ran to my partner, crawled up his chest and tucked herself under his chin. Suffice to say, she came home with us that night. Sleeping on his chest was a connection Squirt maintained for several weeks until, worrying that she was too tired for a young dog,

Figure 5.1: Bramble 'warming' the baby's reusable nappies

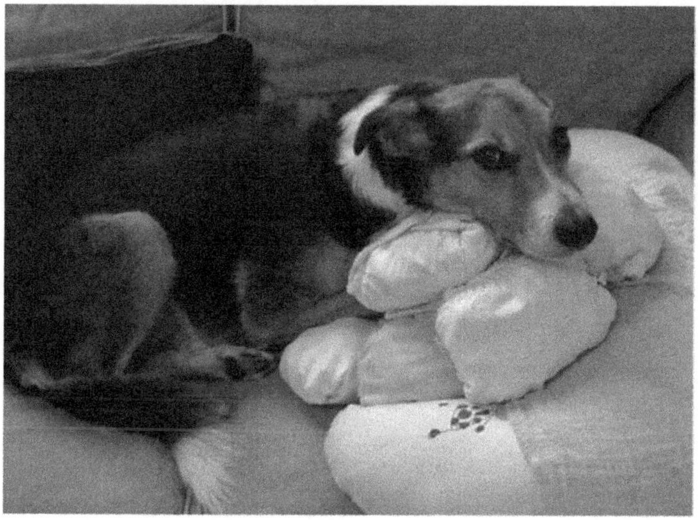

we took her to the vets. The vet recommended neutering her as she was so small and could foresee problems if she were to conceive. During the spay the vet called saying that she was already pregnant, and that the pup was large enough to be a risk to her life. He recommended we abort the pup, and we chose to.

After this Squirt stopped sleeping on my partner's chest, and we wondered why. On bad days, I wonder if it is because we took her reproductive choices away from her, not only by having her neutered but also in choosing to abort her pregnancy. Her patience with our next dog, Loki, as a puppy made me think she would have been wonderful with her own pup (Figure 5.2). Having worked extensively in dog shelters and having seen the heart-rending results of over-populations of domestic dogs, I am – theoretically at least – a proponent of neutering. I do wonder though how we can call them kin, consider them family members and 'persons', yet still wield power over their bodily autonomy (see Armbruster [2010] for a reflection on this).

In this section we have signalled different aspects of kinship, reproduction and normativities. We have highlighted where heteronormativities are troubled in queer family formation, and also where the reproductive potentialities of dogs are delimited. The subsequent behavioural changes in Squirt prompted reflection on autonomy and personhood, a concept often discussed in human-centric dementia studies (for example, Kitwood and Bredin, 1992; Higgs and Gilleard, 2016) and a topic to which we now turn.

Figure 5.2: Squirt showing infinite patience with Loki as a puppy

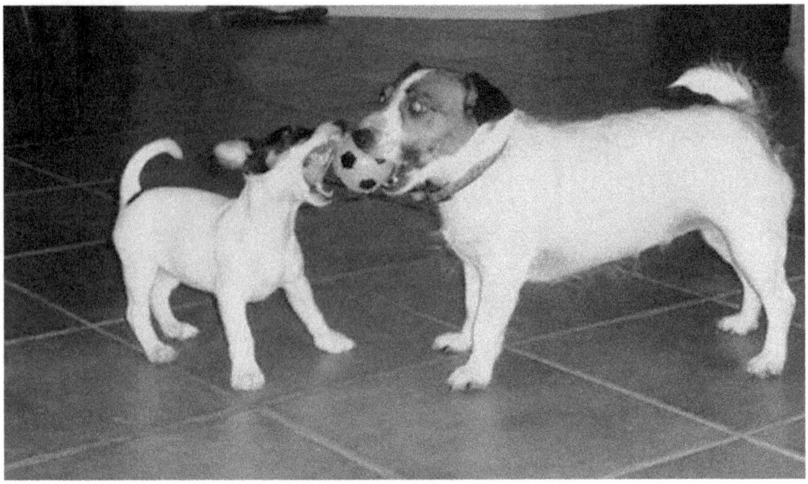

Personhood

In our work on staff in animal shelters (Taylor, 2007), we have argued that central to recognition for animals by staff is the attribution of some form of personhood. This can occur through naming practices (that is, naming animals who come without identification), forming relationships with animals (thus attributing mindedness and agency to animals) and emphasising the perceived personalities of animals. Similar practices of personhood occur in multi-species kinship, where humans and animals together attribute meaning to the relationships that they share (Power, 2008). However, it is worth noting that animal personhood, while considered by many to be a prerequisite for their rights, is flexible. As Shir-Virtesh (2012) in their consideration of pets as family argues, there is a fluidity involved in practices of animal personhood that can be seen as a humanness–animality continuum. In part, the flexibility of the appellation of person to the animals that share our homes reflects human exceptionalism – we get to choose when they belong and should be accorded moral consideration and we equally get to determine when they do not belong and should be discarded (Fox, 2006).

In other words, as we suggested at the beginning of this chapter in regard to love, any attribution of personhood is partial, and contingent on our perceptions about another, as well as dependent upon ideas of family. Charles and Davies (2008), for example, found that those who identified family in terms of blood or marriage were resistant to the idea of pets as family whereas those with more expansive views of family, that also included friends, allowed for the idea of multi-species kinship. Yet such attributions play an important role in multi-species kinship: it helps all parties to form bonds based on shared interests, or concessions to the perceived needs of another, or the mutual fulfillment of relationship needs, such as for affection and company.

Damien: From the beginning Willy lived up to his name. Not only did he have a wonky leg, but a seemingly wonky personality, always doing odd things that made us laugh. Figure 5.3 is a photo of Willy mid-leap, jumping up trying to catch some sparks from an angle grinder. In many ways he was a good match for my eldest child, who himself was something of an odd character. Together they made a good pair, always getting up to no good, with their shared oddness bonding them together. For me, Willy (and my eldest child too) taught me that love and affection can come in odd forms. There was nothing 'dog typical' about Willy (nor 'child typical' about my eldest child). Any assumptions I had about what it would mean to be a parent, or a dog keeper, went out of the window, as I learnt to live with and love these people who were very different to me.

Elizabeth: Bramble was a complex and demanding dog until he slowed down in later life, though he never seemed to fully appreciate that when we had visitors he was not inevitably the focus. Hypervigilant, he needed plenty of mental and physical stimulation for harmonious cohabitation and was destructive in his youth. 'Difficult personalities' make great stories. The eating-the-car-boot-interior-trim tale, and the demolition of the arm of the settee when we were sat next to each other, and many other happenings, are embedded in the family collective memory (Figure 5.4). As Bramble was so bright, we (I) had fly-ball champion, agility whizz and Crufts-ring dog dancing fantasies. Aspirations fulfilled by games of fetch and human–dog kitchen discos. Now having another dog (a rescue Springer Spaniel who is very 'easy') I better understand and appreciate how brilliant and unique he was. Border Collie/terrier crosses are not the next Cockapoo, but he will always be my best in show.

Nik: Squirt was, quite possibly, the biggest small dog I have ever known. Perhaps due to her start in life that involved some time on the streets, she was extremely self-sufficient, at least before her mental decline, and it felt very much like she *chose* to be with us and love us. She was responsive and seemed to like being with us, usually sitting on our knees or on the arm of the couch next to us – and once jumping into the bath with me (Figure 5.5). But she was also extremely stubborn, which felt very much as though she had a wonderfully developed sense of self – she knew who she was and would only do what she wanted. To outsiders this was seen

Figure 5.3: Willy jumping at sparks from an angle grinder

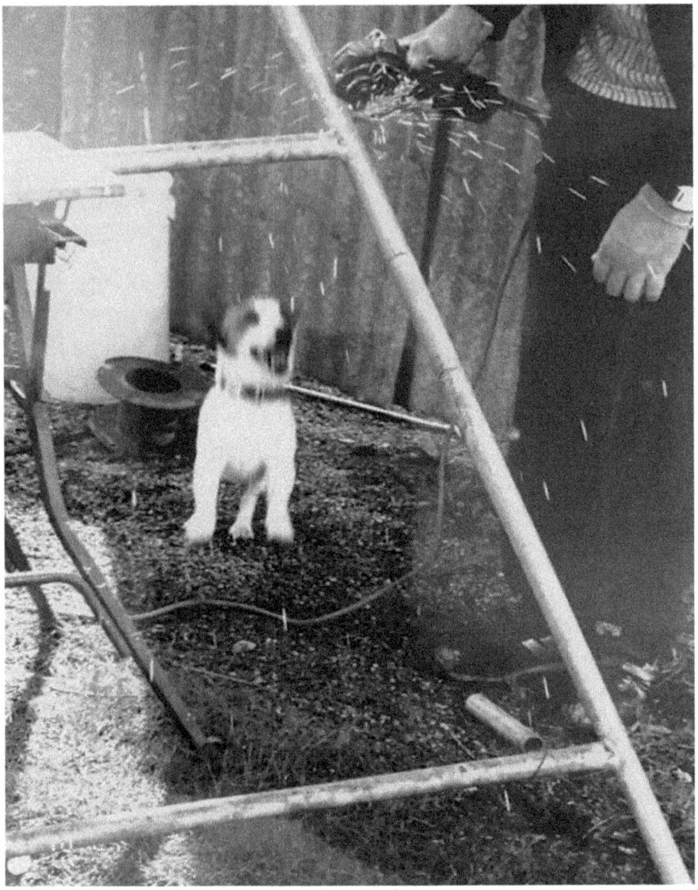

as problematic, but this wilful, stubborn streak really drew me to her and I encouraged it as much as I could, or as much as she would let me. This happened naturally, in response to her personality, but it led to much introspection on my behalf about the way we curtail our companion animal's autonomy. I interact differently with my current dogs – affording them as much choice as is safe within the confines of a human-driven society.

Personhood is a slippery concept when applied to human-centric *and* multi-species ways of being. Though, as Haraway proposes:

> [J]ust *who* is at home must permanently be in question. The recognition that one cannot *know* the other or the self, but must ask in respect for all of time who and what are emerging in relationship, is the key.

> That is so for all true lovers, of whatever species. (Haraway, 2003: 50; original emphasis)

Therefore, as personhood is relational human–dog kinship is shaped by imperfect intersubjectivity, which, as we discuss in what follows, is in flux over time.

The passage of time

Much of the literature on living with animals remarks on the salience of time. Living with animals, for many humans, is marked by awareness that in most instances humans are likely to outlive animals (Garber, 1996). The concept of 'dog years' serves as a way to mark the truncated lifespan of dogs,

Figure 5.4: Bramble with an injured paw that fuelled destructive behaviours as a puppy

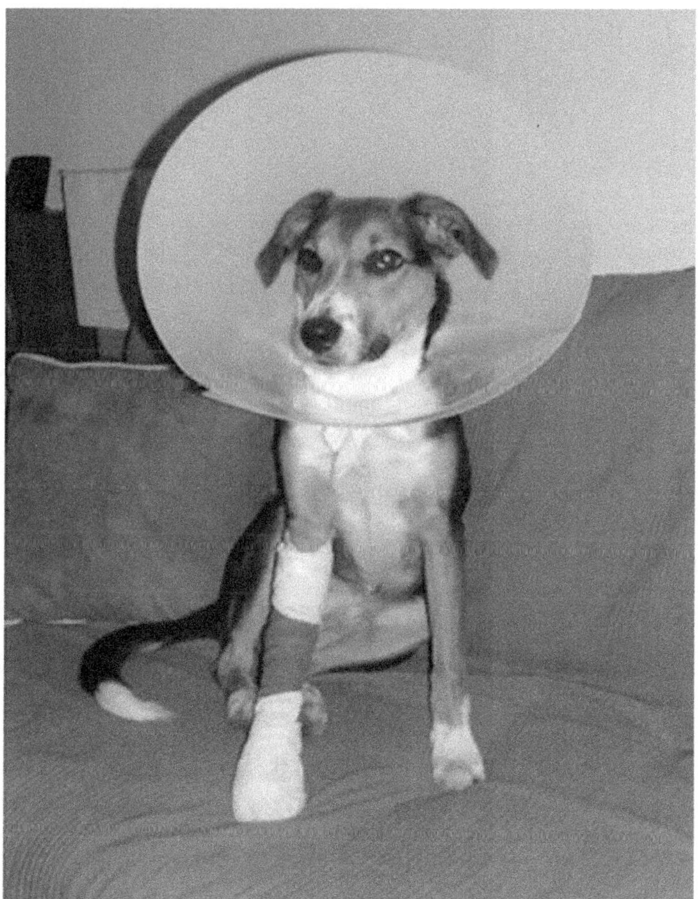

Figure 5.5: Squirt on the couch arm next to us

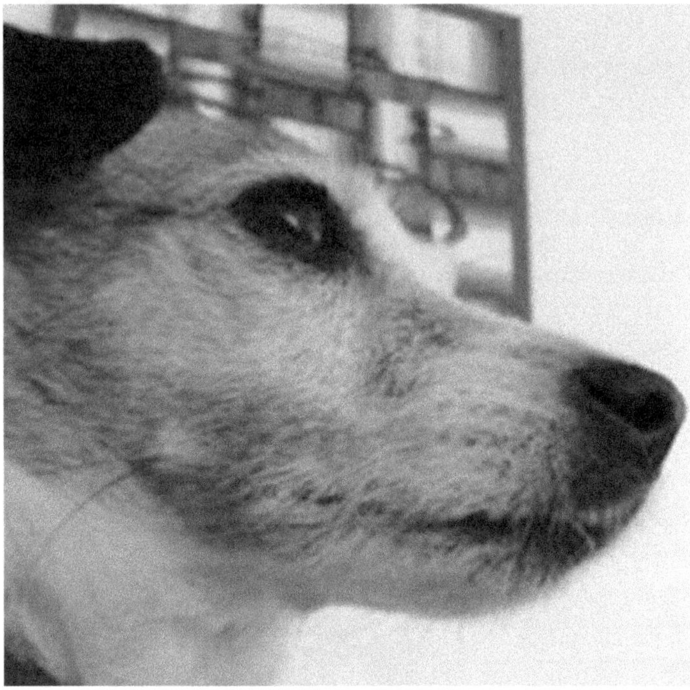

for example, as compared to humans. At the same time, questions have been raised about whether animals themselves mark time at all, let alone in the same fashion as humans (Campbell, 1996). The reduction of animal time to a poor version of human time, however, fundamentally fails to understand animal time as bound by a set of rules that function in similar ways as does human time: animal time, similar to human time, allows for the person to track what is going on in their world, whether that be in relation to food, or safety, or companionship. Animals may not look at a clock, but, especially for domesticated animals, time shapes their lives and in turn guides their actions.

As is true in the case of humans living with dementia, for animals living with dementia the meaning of time changes, and the same is true for their companions. Patterns that were likely well established, such as walk time, or feeding time, or the coming and going of humans, events that might have once evoked much excitement, may change in meaning or cease to have meaning. Further, and as the dementia progresses, human keepers must negotiate the limited time that lies ahead, whether that be by trying to make the most of time available, or by beginning the process of letting go (or both simultaneously). Dementia thus in many ways disrupts the aspects of time that shape human–animal relationships, forcing upon all parties an altered relationship to time, including in terms of routines, and expectations about the future.

Damien: However odd he might have been, Willy always seemed to like routine. He knew when it was bedtime, and made his way straight to his bed, even right to the end when his wonky legs weren't working well. Willy would wait at the door when he knew children were coming home from school, and sometimes reminded me when I was busy working at home that it was time to fetch children from school. Towards the end of his life, however, many of these time-driven aspects of Willy's life appeared to break down. He would forget to eat mid-eating. He would walk in endless circles in the backyard, wearing tracks in the lawn. Because he was such an odd character for all of his life, at first these changes just seemed like a new oddness. In retrospect, I can see he was living with dementia for quite some time before we recognised it.

Elizabeth: Bramble's behavioural and cognitive changes in later life could be attributed to old age or to dementia. Likely his decline was multi-factorial; at 15 years old, as our vet labelled him, he was an 'ancient geriatric'. Age nine he needed first one and then a second cruciate ligament repair which curtailed his running career, but he was an enthusiastic walker for many more years. When we got a second dog when he was 11 that seemed to give him a boost emotionally. He was finally part of a pack which we had always suspected would be beneficial in ameliorating some of his anxieties. His slow physical and mental decline coincided with the COVID-19 pandemic of which the most difficult aspect was the nightly disruption to our sleep. Not sundowning *per se* but barking to be let out two, three or more times a night. We assumed that this behaviour change was a result of old age incontinence. However, during Bramble's last few weeks he would often stand in the garden in the night seemingly confused as to why he was there. If he could have articulated his changed experience perhaps he may have said, like one of my human research participants, 'When you get to eighty-four you DO forget' (Peel, 2015: 1126), normalising his new reality, or perhaps he would have gained a dementia diagnosis.

Nik: Prior to the age of five, when Squirt had her first epileptic fit, she was an outgoing, 'trouble-full', good-natured 'boss' of the house. She taught Loki her manners to such an extent that we barely needed to offer much in the way of training, and she also trained the humans in the household well to give her treats on demand and to install a dog-flap in her house so she had more autonomy. Post-five she began a very slow decline due to us never being able to get her epilepsy under control. This ultimately led to canine cognitive dysfunction which seemed to be both epilepsy- and dementia-based. She slowly withdrew from us, over the next ten years or so, choosing to stay in her extremely large, padded, always open dog cage and rarely interacting with us or the other dogs. To this day, my partner talks about how we were all 'robbed' by the changes in her. With hindsight it's fairly easy to see the slow decline she underwent. But it was so slow that it's impossible pinpoint a certain time and categorically state that this is when she changed, or disappeared from our lives, or that this is when life became unliveable for her. However, disappear she did, and we felt stress and pressure of wondering if we were doing the right thing keeping her going when our daily interactions were simply to give her medication that she loathed and fought us over.

In focusing on the passage of time we have foregrounded the divergent understandings of time from human and canine perspectives, as well as the changing dynamics as dogs age at a faster rate than their human companions. In the remainder of this chapter, we discuss end-of-life decision-making, grief and loss, and in so doing highlight some of the messy and inevitable complexities of multi-species kinship.

Decision-making and social death

The literature on dementia in humans has made use of the concept of 'social death'[9] to refer to the idea that a person can be living at the same time as lacking or having lost the social aspects of their personhood (Sweeting and Gilhooly, 1997; Behuniak, 2011; Peel 2014). Obviously, this account of dementia centres the idea that humans are social animals, and that the loss of sociality is indeed a loss. Moreover, the emphasis upon social death reflects in many ways the loss of a relationship with someone living with dementia: the perceived slipping away of their personhood slowly reduces or removes the standard triggers for the relationship. In the face of perceptions about social death, loved ones must find ways to negotiate new relationships with those living with dementia (Slocombe et al, 2022), at the same time as potentially making decisions on their behalf, particularly when it comes to living arrangements and end-of-life wishes. This may involve attributing 'humanness' to the person – or animal – who has dementia. Bogdan and Taylor (1989) in their now classic consideration of the social construction of humanness outlined how non-disabled people characterise severely disabled people in ways which underline, or construct, their humanity. For example, they attribute thinking to the other, view and act as though the other is reciprocating, and define a social place for them. Additional layers of complexity are added when the person living with dementia is an animal given that human caretakers of healthy dogs often already have to carve out social spaces and personhood for them. As Sanders argues, 'caretakers of companion animals and others who live in everyday situations entailing frequent and intimate interaction with nonhuman animals … consistently see animals as subjective actors and define interactions with them as being "authentic" and reciprocal exchanges' (Sanders, 1993: 206). Yet further complexity is found when human keepers must make decisions about the best interests of animals who cannot easily voice their own wishes (Belshaw et al, 2020).

Damien: Willy's dementia became most noticeable when he started doing things that were, in some respects, anti-social. While he was always an odd dog, he was a very social dog, always wanting to be in the thick of things, always looking for a cuddle. As his dementia progressed Willy spent a lot of time getting into corners and staring at a wall, as can be seen in Figure 5.6. I would leave a room and come back to find him stuck under a chair staring at nothing, or wedged in the corner of a room against furniture, not moving. At first this often made us chuckle, but over time it created an odd gap between us and Willy. Gone was the funny, engaging, caring person we had lived with for well over a decade, and instead there was this odd figure or facsimile of Willy. He still looked mostly the same (even if a lot older), but his presence had changed: from a loved family member to a person almost akin to an object in the room. It was the loss of the relationship with him that crept up on us slowly.

These changes in Willy's personhood led my mother to ask what were Willy's best interests. With his growing disinterest in food (or at least remembering to eat it), and his disengagement from us as family members, she asked what his quality of life was. For me, as much as things had changed so much with Willy, it was hard to imagine our family without him. He had been there from early on in raising my first child, and was still there four children later. I struggled with whether I was being selfish wanting him to be with us, and not seeing many signs that life was inherently unhappy for him. The weight of making a decision, and in the context of having children who would miss him terribly, was one that I sat with for a long period of time, coaxing Willy (with the help of our vet) through the loss (and regaining) of the use of his back lags, his loss of appetite, and his loss of orientation to the space around him. Medication certainly helped address some of these issues, though omnipresent was the feeling that, ultimately, we would have to make a decision about Willy's life.

Elizabeth: Despite his advanced years and frailty Bramble did, on reflection, have a 'good' quality of life until his last few weeks. As is shown in Figure 5.7 he was included in family holidays. He was stoic and never

Figure 5.6: Willy facing the wall

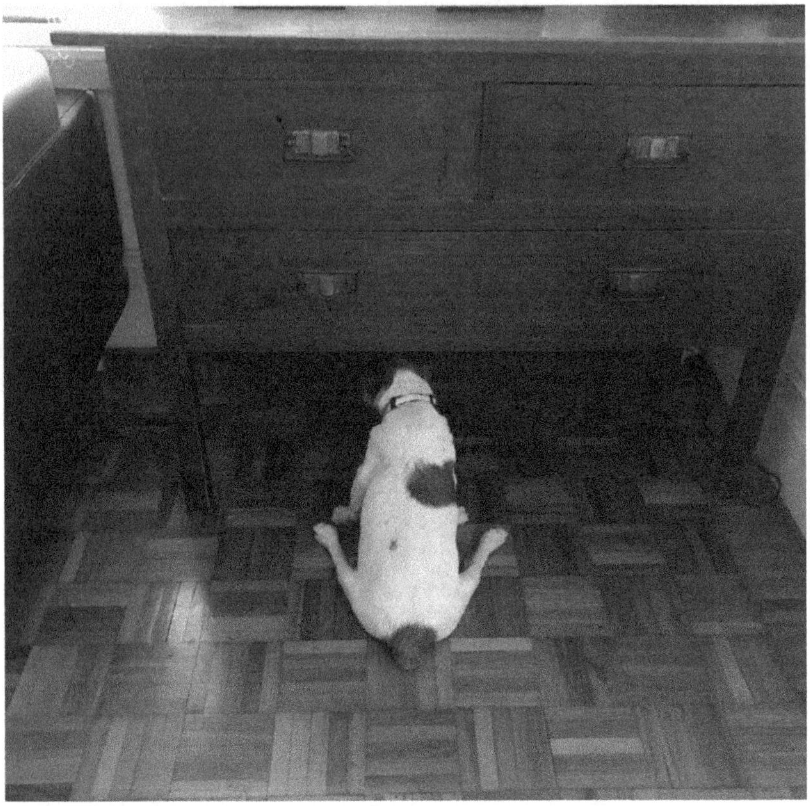

refused to walk or embrace the moment – even if he was clearly exhausted by it all. In retrospect, we should perhaps have been more Bramble-centred and scaled back, though he did not now venture upstairs and largely slept when not walking. When left to his own devices he was withdrawn, no longer a willing or able dance partner. And he rarely wagged his tail – all signs that life was increasingly challenging. But he was a healthy, fit animal and could walk, albeit steadily, some considerable distance quite close to the end of his life. When we checked in with the vet his view was an optimistic one, the arthritis medications Bramble had taken for many years weren't interfering with his liver function and his hearing and vision were still largely intact. Despite human optimism and a can-do approach, it was the other animals in the home who began to indicate his deteriorating state. Our cat, who had regularly play-fought with Bramble, now kept a respectful distance, and our other dog Poppy – the more dominant dog – started making concessions and let him actually have his toys. In multi-species kinship noticing cues from all loved ones

Figure 5.7: Bramble frail and sleeping in the sunshine on one of his last holidays

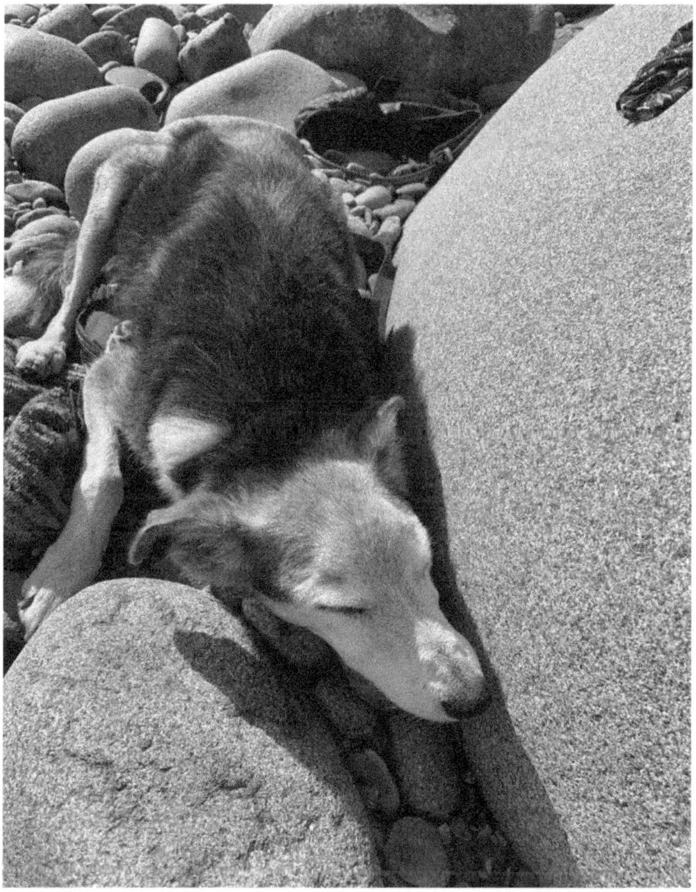

is part of the landscape. Haraway (2003: 41) wrote that 'inter-subjectivity does not mean "equality", a literally deadly game in dogland; but it does mean paying attention to the conjoined dance of face-to-face significant otherness'. The tenor and form of the dance in our family was shifting as the animals slowly withdrew from Bramble, and Bramble withdrew from us all.

Nik: As mentioned earlier, Squirt slowly withdrew from us which would seem to make the decision about the end of her life easier, yet it didn't. Physically, she was still robust and healthy. Our vet in fact, a week or so before she died, said her blood work was that of an eight-year-old dog (she was 15 at the time), which made our decision-making process all the harder. But her withdrawal from us actually made the decision harder for me. She seemed so inwardly focused on her own illness and this, combined with her

Figure 5.8: Squirt, tired post-fit

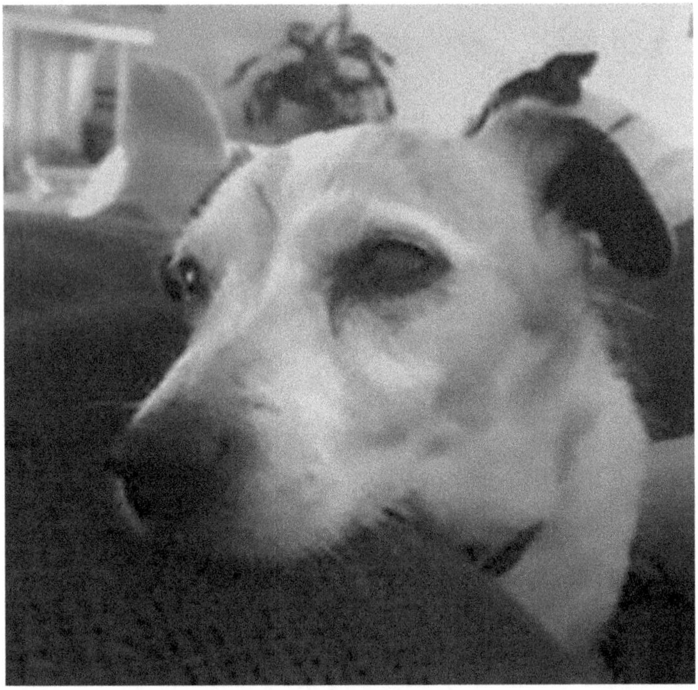

self-removal from our social sphere, made it hard for me to read her (Figure 5.8). I missed her presence, to be sure, but I also missed being able to check in with her through touching her, or asking her questions and watching her response, and this added complexity to the decision of whether to euthanise her or not. Towards the very end, I also started to question if I was thinking of euthanising her because of the impact her illness had on our quality of life, which was considerable: we were sleep-deprived due to her nightly wakefulness, we wouldn't leave the house for more than a few hours at a time in case she had a fit while we were out, holidays were impossible – we had tried taking her with us on one and her panic at being removed from her safe spaces meant we came home the next day, we had weekly vet visits that we had to fit in around work and I started with terrible insomnia due to constantly berating myself for not doing enough for her. All of this made the decision to euthanise her extremely complex and difficult – far more so than I have ever faced with other dogs.

Grieving

Connected to the concept of social death is the concept of ambiguous loss (Boss, 2000). Ambiguous loss refers to a loss that may be unresolved due to, for example, a person or dog who is missing (that is, not knowing if they are still alive) (Allen et al, 2022), or in the case of dementia, someone who is physically present but psychologically absent for an extended period of time (Dupuis, 2002). As a result, grieving the person after their death can be fraught by the often substantive changes to our relationship with them prior to their death. Ambiguous loss is equally applicable to animals living with dementia as it is to humans living with dementia, but is likely compounded by what Laing and Maylea (2018: 223) refer to as 'anthropocentrically disenfranchised grief'. The loss of an animal may be disenfranchised when other humans do not recognise the loss as valid, or do not appreciate the depth and extent of grief associated with the death of an animal (Meyers, 2002). Redmalm (2015) argues that to a certain extent the death of an animal is commonly framed in Western cultures as less-than-grieveable for three reasons. First, grief is often premised on the idea of irreplaceability (that is, the lost person cannot be substituted for another), yet too often animals are treated in Western cultures in general as objects that are easily replaced (or indeed consumed). Second, grief is a product of the relationship with the person who is gone, yet too often animals are seen as lacking the personhood necessary to constitute a relationship. Third, grief is commonly an embodied experience: both felt within the body, but also involving the loss of the body of another. Again, when animals are all too often reduced to mere bodies (for the purpose of human consumption and/or benefit), seeing the loss of an animal as evoking a visceral human response is often treated as less than intelligible.

Of course, this focuses on whether human grief for an animal following dementia is seen as intelligible. But what of animal grief? How do animals grieve for one another? If recognition of human grief is disenfranchised, then animal grief is rarely acknowledged at all (Pribac, 2021). As we have explored elsewhere (Riggs and Peel, 2016), however, animals often display considerable grief responses when a companion dies: whether that be a human keeper or animal kin. What has rarely been given attention, however, is how animals appear to make sense of animal kin living with dementia, and what that means for their grief.

Damien: At the very end of his life, Willy had forgotten how to toilet outside, had seemingly forgotten who we all were (both humans and other animals), and was struggling to remember to eat. This created a lot of work for me, having to clean up waste, lift him up to toilet, find him when he got lost outside, and to try and coax him to eat (including buying roast chicken to try and entice him, which constituted another struggle for me as a vegan). My mother continued to advocate for the 'humane option', but I struggled to say goodbye. I think in many ways my children had already said goodbye, given Willy had been distant for so long. One day I woke up and Willy was struggling to stand at all. This was on a day I was to present at a conference on animals and death. Cancelling my presentation, I sat with and held Willy for the final hours of his life. Time was of the essence, as I knew the children would be home later that day, and I wanted for Willy to be in his final resting place before they returned. But I also wanted to enjoy my final moments with this wonky, odd dog. Our other dogs came in for a sniff and left again, but Willy was not aware of their presence. They too seemed to have already accepted that he was gone. In his final moments I reflected on how thankful I was to have known Willy, how much he had given our family, and how little he had asked for in return.

In many ways, the death of Willy was treated as intelligible in my broader family. I think this was largely due to the fact that we had previously gone through the death of a dog who had been my very close companion, and for whom I had experienced significant grief. One of my children had also experienced considerable grief when another dog had died suddenly. These previous deaths had, I think, primed my extended family to be mindful of the grief we would likely experience when Willy died. Yet given the extended period of social death we had lived through, Willy's passing was in many ways a relief, and for me in particular, relief that I had not had to end his life. Nonetheless, I was thankful that other people asked about him, and checked in with how I was going. While my grief for Willy might have been different to grief for other animals, he had still been part of my family for a long time. To know that others saw his personhood and thus understand he was missed, was important.

Elizabeth: We had numerous soul-searching moments and difficult conversations on the run up to euthanising Bramble. Although his mobility and memory were now curtailed, he was still eating and drinking but losing weight and increasingly wobbly on his feet. Uncertainty around 'curbside' pandemic veterinary care loomed large in our thinking too. When we had taken Bramble to have an end-of-life conversation with a vet from the boot of the car, there was a man sobbing in the carpark. He'd evidently just handed over his dog; we had to be there for Bramble but this was far from guaranteed given the restrictions in place at the time. I found a home pet euthanasia service which was still operating, and when the day came we asked our now ten-year-old child to say her goodbyes as he would not be there when she returned from school.

During an agonising day tensioning animal and human care I spoke with 'dignivets' who didn't have capacity to come that day, the crematorium and our local vet. I persuaded our vet to bend the rules and we were able to comfort Bramble while in his bed in the boot of the car, reversed surreptitiously down to the back entrance of the practice. Through the grief there will always be gratitude that we were able to be with him at a time when so many were separated from their loved ones at the end of life. It was important to us that all members of the family got to 'say goodbye' so enroute to the crematorium we drove Bramble home. Frodo the cat sniffed his body, ran away and was seemingly unperturbed. In Poppy, however, there was evidence of physical and emotional distress for some weeks. She was disinterested in food and had digestive problems, and she seemed maudlin and listless. They loved him too.

Nik: When Squirt died we lived with two other dogs, Loki and Bailey. So far as I could tell neither of them showed any real grief. I had expected they might, based on prior experiences of other dogs losing their kin, but I believe Squirt's slow removal of herself from our spheres meant that she had already been grieved over. This was certainly the case for me. The day we spoke to the vet about putting her down the next day, he asked if we wanted a few days to work through our grief with her and I replied 'I have been grieving this dog for ten years'. And while losing her was awful – as it always is, and is still raw enough now that even three years later, writing this chapter was a real struggle – her actual death was perhaps the 'easiest' I've experienced due, again, to this slow withdrawal of her from our lives.

Conclusion

In thinking about living with and grieving for animals who have dementia, in this chapter we have emphasised a critical kinship studies framework to highlight the importance of focusing on loss and love in multi-species households. We have also utilised a queer menagerie approach to bring our own stories together with the literature on animals, dementia and death, with the aim of contributing to how we think about the loss of an animal to dementia. What has been on display has been our own human processes of living with dementia, as well as our representations of Bramble, Willy and Squirt's personhood as we understand them. While acknowledging the partiality of any experience of love and the personhood of another, our hope has been to signal the importance of at least trying to think about what animal dementia means not just for humans, but for animals themselves, including the companions of those living with dementia. What might we learn by decentring dementia as a solely human experience and increasing focus on how canine dementia experiences pattern human–animal kinship in both life and in death? On one reading this chapter has simply been an act of memorialisation and legacy-giving to our much-loved dogs. On another reading, there may be potentialities for a more thoroughgoing queering of understandings of dementia (Shildrick, 2021) by being attentive to speciesism and foregrounding other species' experiences alongside our human ones.

In many ways our stories shared in this chapter reflect the literature on the loss of an animal (for example, Satama and Huopalainen, 2019; Morris, 2020). Even though as humans we enter into relationships with animals knowing they are unlikely to outlive us, and in the case of dementia, knowing that at some point in the near future our loved one will be gone, this knowledge does not automatically equate to preparedness. We can know something in our mind, but to know it in our heart is another matter entirely. Certainly, in some of our stories we found ourselves pulling away from an animal living with dementia, or found that they pulled away from us. This potentially gives us some space for which to prepare for impending loss and grief. But the actual embodied, experiential aspects of grief are much harder to prepare for. Even if we have been distanced from someone due to dementia, their death still leaves a hole, and it is only after death that we begin to feel the shape and size of that hole.

Grief and the shape it takes may be further compounded by the end-of-life decisions humans sometimes have to make when it comes to animals. Certainly, the idea of a 'just death' is as equally applicable to animals as it is to humans (Sanders, 1995), even if cultures of animal consumption might often serve to sideline the personhood of animals and their right to life and to a just death. But at the same time, we must consider on what basis humans can make decisions about what constitutes quality of life for an animal, and thus what constitutes a just death. As some of our stories highlight, animal dementia is often accompanied by high levels of emotional and physical labour for humans (Belshaw et al, 2020). Is it possible to separate out the decisions we make about a just death for an animal from our own needs (that is, to provide palliative care, to witness suffering)? At the same time, we might argue that making end-of-life decisions reflect the nature of the relationship: that responsibility for another's life reflects our love for them and their trust and love for us. It is likely that there is no one pathway to decision-making, but rather that it reflects the intersections of human and animal needs, responsibility, and the rights of animals to a just death.

The limited number of publications specifically on animals living with dementia (for example, Anderson, 2016) often pay little attention to the complex and fraught nature of living with dementia in multi-species households. Instead, the focus is often on the pragmatic, emphasising care routines, healthcare and end-of-life decisions. In this literature the focus tends to be on how humans experience disenfranchised grief at the loss of an animal, with little in-depth focus on the complexities of human grief for an animal lost to dementia in a broader world where grief for animals is so often seen as less than intelligible. Similarly, there is little focus on the animals themselves beyond welfarist driven debates about the practical aspects of their quality of life: whether, how and in what ways they experience their illness and (perceived) decline is left unconsidered. In part, this may be due to the impracticalities of knowing how other animals think, but it is also part of our humanist legacy wherein we remain fixated on human processes and understandings. A critical kinship studies focus on multi-species households, by contrast, centres love and emotions, and recognises the queer menageries created by humans and animals together. Into the future, then, needed are approaches to the topic that engage in diverse ways of thinking through what dementia means to both humans and animals. As we have noted from the beginning of this chapter, while love may always be partial, that does not mean that as humans we should not do our level best to at least try to understand and represent the meaning of dementia for animals, both for those living with dementia, and for animals who lose a companion to dementia.

Animal psychologists note that 'cute dogs, with baby-like features, tend to be preferred as pets and are treated more humanely by their owners' (Piazza, 2020: 122), which raises important questions for the place of the older dog with dementia in nexuses of care. While Bramble, for example, was labelled an 'ancient geriatric' by his vet, there was no discussion of his behaviour being indicative of dementia, or discussion of possible treatment of symptoms. Should veterinary professionals be seen, in this context, as embedded in the critical kinship nexus with skills to bear in managing expectations of both their canine and human clients? Expectations not solely focused on end-of-life decision-making but also on naming and claiming canine cognitive dysfunction and working in collaboration with human household members to maximise enabling the animal to live well.[10] This may be an idealistic aspiration given how veterinary medicine is structured and the financial pressures on many pet owners, however, opening space in consultations for dementia-related conversations alongside destigmatising canine cognitive dysfunction in veterinary practice could yield benefits for non-humans and humans alike.

Acknowledgements

Thanks to Jamie Arathoon and the editors for their helpful feedback on an earlier version of this chapter.

Notes

1 The editors drew our attention to the possibility that our chapter may 'qualify' as a piece of post-qualitative inquiry, which 'encourages concrete, practical experimentation and the creation of the not yet instead of the repetition of what is' (St Pierre, 2019: 3). We had not considered this prior to this being raised, however, we are open to this possibility given '[p]ost qualitative inquiry does not exist prior to its arrival; it must be created, invented anew each time. [And it] begins with an encounter with the real, not with method' (St Pierre, 2019: 9, 11). Gough (2021: 4) remarks that post-qualitative enquiry can 'disrupt human intentions, practices and projects. It is the nonhuman which is afforded agency', and in keeping with foregrounding the non-human we

have endeavoured to prioritise our canine companions in the experiential account that follows.

2 Acknowledging that we each as humans have very different experiences of animal companionship, and that our experiences of living with another's dementia also differ.

3 We do not suggest that photographs 'give voice' to each of them, but photographs do at the very least bring Bramble, Willy and Squirt into the story in a different medium. Moreover, we designedly chose images of our dogs on their own, rather than with us or other humans, to foreground them visibly in the text and convey a sense of them as an embodied being with a dementia trajectory in the absence of being able to access their perspectives via a different lens or mechanism. This choice to exclude us shouldn't be interpreted as our minimising the relational contexts and interactions we had with our dogs.

4 This focus on messiness is deliberate, an ongoing reminder of the need to disrupt the 'purification power game' (Taylor, 2012: 42) that sees humans and other animals as ontologically and epistemologically distinct – a power game that allows us to wilfully exclude other animals from 'the social', from our spheres of concern.

5 Pronatalism is policies and practices which encourage people to have children, and as we've suggested elsewhere, 'the cultural expectation of pronatalism becomes naturalized, so much so that having children is seen as "natural", with not having children seen as "unnatural"' (Riggs and Peel, 2016: 37).

6 And often particular forms of human–human kinship. Strathern (1992b: 19) in the context of British kinship highlighted that 'nature has increasingly come to mean biology'. Critique of the place and status of genetic relatedness in kinship is a key constituent of critical kinship studies.

7 Though characterising Bramble in human kinship terms, we align with Haraway's observation that 'contrary to lots of dangerous and unethical projection in the Western world that makes domestic canines into furry children, dogs are not about oneself. Indeed, that is the beauty of dogs. They are not a projection, nor the realization of an intention, nor the telos of anything. They are dogs, i.e., a species in obligatory, constitutive, historical, protean relationship with human beings. … To regard a dog as a furry child, even metaphorically, demeans dogs and children' (2003: 10–11, 37).

8 In retrospect what were evidently legitimate worries about Bramble harming the baby were overblown, likely exacerbated by the loss of my first pregnancy (Peel and Cain, 2012).

9 It is important to recognise that latterly there have been counters to this form of deficit narrative through supported self-advocacy and activism from people living with dementia (for example, see Weetch et al, 2021), and the concept of social death is also ableist in that reduced cognitive function is linked with death.

10 For instance, discussion in veterinary consultations about the health and wellbeing benefits of dog walking could be beneficial for both parties (Reynolds, 2022; cf Peel et al, 2010).

References

Allen, D., Arathoon, J. and Selby-Fell, H. (2022) 'Experiences of dog theft and spatial practices of search/ing', *The Geographical Journal*, 188(4): 518–533.

Anderson, E. (2016) *Remember Me? Loving and Caring for a Dog with Canine Cognitive Dysfunction*, Washington, DC: Dogwise Publishing.

Armbruster, K. (2010) 'Into the wild: Response, respect, and the human control of canine sexuality and reproduction', *JAC*, 30(3/4): 755–783.

Behuniak, S.M. (2011) 'The living dead? The construction of people with Alzheimer's disease as zombies', *Ageing & Society*, 31(1): 70–92.

Belshaw, Z., Dean, R. and Asher, L. (2020) '"You can be blind because of loving them so much": The impact on owners in the United Kingdom of living with a dog with osteoarthritis', *BMC Veterinary Research*, 16(1): 1–10.

Bogdan, R. and Taylor, S. (1989) 'Relationships with severely disabled people: The social construction of humanness', *Social Problems*, 36(2): 135–148.

Boss, P. (2000) *Ambiguous Loss: Learning to Live with Unresolved Grief*, Cambridge, MA: Harvard University Press.

Campbell, J. (1996) 'Human vs animal time', in M.A Pastor and J. Artieda (eds) *Time, Internal Clocks and Movement*, Amsterdam: Elsevier, pp 115–126.

Charles, N. and Davies, C. (2008) 'My family and other animals: Pets as kin', *Sociological Research Online*, 13(5): 13–26.

Dupuis, S.L. (2002) 'Understanding ambiguous loss in the context of dementia care: Adult children's perspectives', *Journal of Gerontological Social Work*, 37(2): 93–115.

Ellis, S.J., Riggs, D.W. and Peel, E. (2020) *Lesbian, Gay, Bisexual, Trans, Intersex and Queer Psychology: An Introduction*, 2nd edn, Cambridge: Cambridge University Press.

Fox, R. (2006) 'Animal behaviours, post-human lives: Everyday negotiations of the animal–human divide in pet-keeping', *Social & Cultural Geography*, 7(4): 525–537.

Garber, M. (1996) *Dog Love*, New York, NY: Touchstone.

Gillespie, K. (2022) 'For multispecies autoethnography', *Environment and Planning E: Nature and Space*, 5(4): 2098–2111.

Gough, B. (2021) 'Imagining a vibrant [post]qualitative psychology via "experimentation"', *Methods in Psychology*, 4: 100049.

Hamilton, L. and Taylor, N. (2017) *Ethnography After Humanism: Power, Politics and Method in Multi-Species Research*, London: Palgrave.

Haraway, D. (2003) *The Companions Species Manifesto: Dogs, People, and Significant Others*, Chicago, IL: Prickly Paradigm Press.

Higgs, P. and Gilleard, C. (2016) 'Interrogating personhood and dementia', *Aging & Mental Health*, 20(8): 773–780.

Huopalainen, A. (2022) Writing with the bitches. *Organization*, 29(6), 959–978.

Kitwood, T. and Bredin, K. (1992) 'Towards a theory of dementia care: Personhood and well-being', *Ageing and Society*, 12(3): 269–287.

Laing, M. and Maylea, C. (2018) '"They burn brightly, but only for a short time": The role of social workers in companion animal grief and loss', *Anthrozoös*, 31(2): 221–232.

Landsberg, G.M., Nichol, J. and Araujo, J.A. (2012) 'Cognitive dysfunction syndrome: A disease of canine and feline brain aging', *Veterinary Clinics: Small Animal Practice*, 42(4): 749–768.

McHugh, S. (2012) 'Bitch, bitch, bitch: Personal criticism, feminist theory, and dog-writing', *Hypatia*, 27(3): 616–635.

Meyers, B. (2002) 'Disenfranchised grief and the loss of an animal companion', in K.J. Doka (ed) *Disenfranchised Grief: New Directions, Challenges, and Strategies for Practice*, Champaign, IL: Research Press, pp 251–264.

Morris, B. (2020) 'Love and horror in grief: An autopsychography on the loss of a beloved animal companion', *Journal of Humanistic Psychology*, 64(1): 64–78.

Peel, E. (2014) '"The living death of Alzheimer's" versus "Take a walk to keep dementia at bay": Representations of dementia in print media and carer discourse', *Sociology of Health and Illness*, 36(6): 885–901.

Peel, E. (2015) 'Diagnostic communication in the memory clinic: A conversation analytic perspective', *Aging & Mental Health*, 19(12): 1123–1130.

Peel, E. and Cain, R. (2012) 'Silent miscarriage and deafening heteronormativity: A British experiential and critical feminist account', in S. Earle, C. Komaromy and L.L. Layne (eds) *Understanding Reproductive Loss: Perspectives on Life, Death and Fertility*, London: Routledge, pp 79–92.

Peel, E., Douglas, M., Parry, O. and Lawton, J. (2010) 'Type 2 diabetes and dog walking: Patients' longitudinal perspectives about implementing and sustaining physical activity', *British Journal of General Practice*, 60(577): 570–577.

Piazza, J. (2020) 'Why people love animals yet continue to eat them', in K. Dhont and G. Hodson (eds) *Why We Love and Exploit Animals: Bringing Insights from Academia and Activism*, London: Routledge, pp 121–136.

Power, E. (2008) 'Furry families: Making a human–dog family through home', *Social & Cultural Geography*, 9(5): 535–555.

Pribac, T.B. (2021) *Enter the Animal: Cross-Species Perspectives on Grief and Spirituality*, Sydney: Sydney University Press.

Redmalm, D. (2015) 'Pet grief: When is non-human life grievable?', *The Sociological Review*, 63(1): 19–35.

Reti, I. and Sien, S. (eds) (1991) *Cats (and their Dykes): An Anthology*, Santa Cruz, CA: HerBooks.

Reynolds, G. (2022) 'Dogs and humans both can get dementia: More walks can help', *The Washington Post*, 16 November. Available from: https://www.washingtonpost.com/wellness/2022/11/16/dogs-dementia-exercise/ [Accessed 22 November 2022].

Riggs, D.W. and Peel, E. (2016) *Critical Kinship Studies: An Introduction to the Field*, Basingstoke: Palgrave Macmillan.

Riggs, D.W., Rosenberg, S., Fraser, H. and Taylor, N. (2021) *Queer Entanglements: Intersections of Gender, Sexuality, and Animal Companionship*, Cambridge: Cambridge University Press.

Sanders, C. (1993) 'Understanding dogs: Caretakers' attributions of mindedness in canine-human relationships', *Journal of Contemporary Ethnography*, 22(2): 205–226.

Sanders, C.R. (1995) 'Killing with kindness: Veterinary euthanasia and the social construction of personhood', *Sociological Forum*, 10(2): 195–214.

Satama, S. and Huopalainen, A. (2019) '"Please tell me when you are in pain": A heartbreaking story of care, grief and female–canine companionship', *Gender, Work & Organization*, 26(3): 358–376.

Shildrick, M. (2021) 'Queering dementia: Technologies, visceral prostheses and embodiment', *Lambda Nordica*, 26(2–3): 76–101.

Shir-Vertesh, D. (2012) '"Flexible personhood": Loving animals as family members in Israel', *American Anthropologist*, 114(3): 420–432.

Slocombe, F., Peel, E., Pilnick, A. and Albert, S. (2022) 'Keeping the conversation going: How progressivity is prioritised in co-remembering talk between couples impacted by dementia', *Health*, 28(2): 272–289.

St Pierre, E. (2019) 'Post qualitative inquiry in an ontology of immanence', *Qualitative Inquiry*, 25(1): 3–16.

Strathern, M. (1992a) *Reproducing the Future: Anthropology, Kinship, and the New Reproductive Technologies*, Manchester: Manchester University Press.

Strathern, M. (1992b) *After Nature: English Kinship in the Late Twentieth Century*, Cambridge: Cambridge University Press.

Sutton, Z. (2020) 'Researching towards a critically posthumanist future: On the political "doing" of critical research for companion animal liberation', *International Journal of Sociology and Social Policy*, 41(3/4): 376–390.

Sweeting, H. and Gilhooly, M. (1997) 'Dementia and the phenomenon of social death', *Sociology of Health & Illness*, 19(1): 93–117.

Taylor, N. (2007) '"Never an it": Intersubjectivity and the creation of animal personhood in animal shelters', *Qualitative Sociology Review*, 3(1): 59–73.

Taylor, N. (2012) 'Animals, mess, method: Post-humanism, sociology and animal studies', in L. Birke and J. Hockenhull (eds) *Crossing Boundaries: Investigating Human Animal Relationships*, Boston, MA: Brill, pp 37–50.

Weetch, J., O'Dwyer, S. and Clare, L (2021) 'The involvement of people with dementia in advocacy: A systematic narrative review', *Aging & Mental Health*, 25(9): 1595–1604.

Wolfe, C. (2010) *What Is Posthumanism?* Minnesota: University of Minneapolis Press.

6

End-of-life entanglements during the COVID-19 lockdowns: caring for and caring about human and non-human animals

Vanessa Ashall

Introduction

In this chapter I share my own interspecies family experiences of dementia, end-of-life care and bereavement. I describe how my experiences during the COVID-19 lockdowns helped me to explore and distinguish the concepts of caring for and caring about both humans and non-human animals at the end of their lives. I highlight the extent to which these concepts shape and separate contemporary landscapes in veterinary and medical understandings of end-of-life care. First, I explore the historic loss of an aged pet and the subsequent realisation that my dog would have lived longer in lockdown. I describe how being relieved of the daily responsibilities which had prevented me from continuing to care for him prompted me to separate the emotional (caring about) and physical (caring for) aspects of veterinary euthanasia decision-making. I show how these concepts may be important for understanding the guilt commonly associated with the euthanasia of loved non-human family members. Next, I describe the experience of being unable to visit a family member who was living with dementia in a care home during the weeks leading up to their death. I share my guilt and distress at being prevented from any physical touch or meaningful conversation due to the COVID-19 lockdown. I show how I came to rely on what I had learnt from the loss of my pet to deal with my guilt and grief: That being prevented from a role in caring for my relative need not correspond to any measure of how much I cared about them. Finally, I consider the clinical implications of our capacities to care for and care about both humans and non-human animals at the end of their lives. I outline the pathophysiological parallels which are drawn between species in chronic neurodegenerative disease and the paradigmatic differences between the clinical treatment of human and non-human animals. I ask to what extent these differences will be tested by increasing efforts to care for ageing animals through the transfer of clinical practices between medical and veterinary settings. Finally, this chapter illustrates the value of thinking across the care of human and non-human species to broadening our understanding of the meanings of care at the end of a life, and engages with speculative interests in caring relationships between humans and non-human animals.

In this chapter I interweave my lived experiences of loss, grief and guilt with observations on veterinary euthanasia practices, analysis of existing theoretical work on concepts of care and interspecies entanglements, and my vision for a speculative future in end-of-life care. In line with recent descriptions of post-qualitative inquiry, my goal is thus 'not to find and represent something that exists in the empirical world of human lived experience but to re-orient thought to experiment and create new forms of thought and life' (St Pierre, 2021: 163). That is not to say that my arguments are not grounded in reality, indeed, my use of personal experience as a lens through which to examine and/or critique cultural experience is well-recognised within autoethnographic research (Adams et al, 2016). What I wish to present here, through bringing into conversation these different forms of knowledge about care at the end of a life, is a provocation for us to think differently, beyond species boundaries, about what caring for those living with dementia *could* mean.

My dog would have lived longer in lockdown

I was standing in the supermarket when I realised that my dog was going to be put to sleep that day. He was at home, asleep as always at that time, and I was filling my basket with anything that I thought might tempt him to eat: sausages; cheese; nothing that a dog really should be eating. The realisation crashed over me like a wave while I stood in the checkout queue that even if I managed to tempt him to eat a morsel of cheese, that I would still not be able to travel to London for work the following day as he would need to be helped out to the garden every hour. Even if I allowed my friend to take on this task again, I would not be able to leave him to go away with my husband and children for a family seventieth birthday celebration that weekend. It dawned on me that I could not hold on to the dog I loved any longer, not because he was any sicker than he had been the day before, but because I could no longer look after him properly.

Stunned by my realisation, I robotically bought the food I had chosen for him. It would have felt barbaric to contemplate putting it back. On the tearful drive home my shocking decision rapidly developed into a surprisingly practical plan: I calculated that we would all need some time to recover from the trauma of losing Snoopy before the family party, that I wanted to let Snoopy go while we were alone in the house and the kids were still at school, but that I needed my husband to come home early to help us all bury him in the garden. I even acknowledged that the sausages would come in handy for the kids' tea if I was too upset to cook.

When I got home I moved into action mode, bravely made the necessary calls, put the plan in motion and then lay down in a patch of sun on the carpet with Snoopy to wait for the vet to arrive. I felt strangely calm. Everything went as it should and Snoopy went to sleep quietly in my arms, but the second his body went limp I knew that I had been wrong. I should have kept trying with the cheese, taken sick leave from work and cancelled the family birthday plans because I loved him and I wasn't ready to lose him. Already, I would have sacrificed anything to spend just one more day with him. Already, I could not comprehend how I could have made that decision, I felt that I had let him down, that I had not loved him enough.

Caring for and caring about animals

Although I am a vet myself, and perhaps also because of this, my feelings of guilt and regret over choosing to let Snoopy go on that day have stayed with me for many years. I now have another young dog who kept me and my family company through the COVID-19 lockdowns, but I thought of Snoopy then more than ever. Like all other households across the UK and beyond, in 2020 our lives were turned upside down as we stopped going to work, stopped going to school and stopped seeing our friends and family. All of these crucial parts of our lives disappeared overnight due to the lockdowns and against this backdrop and the new space to think that it brought, a small but troubling thought started developing in my mind.

I was in the garden during that hot endless spring of the first 2020 lockdown, with nowhere to go, no one to see and my whole family were compelled to stay at home, desperately trying to think of something useful to do. I remember the sun shining through the branches of the tree beneath which Snoopy is buried and the sound of the leaves moving gently in the barely existent breeze as my constantly anxious mind wandered, and I allowed myself to think of him again. Like a thunderbolt, just as had happened in the supermarket, the realisation came to me that I would not have made that same decision today. I was stunned to realise that despite the death and the heartache that we were all experiencing and observing daily, my beloved Snoopy would undoubtedly have lived longer in lockdown.

During lockdown I could have spent all my time with Snoopy and taken care of him in ways which were impossible at the time he died. I could have given him small amounts of food all day long and taken him out to the garden every hour. I could have sat with him every day and stroked him while he slept at my feet. I could have made his life bearable, and made his life possible, now that all the other pressures I usually faced in my life had been removed. I saw even more clearly now that the reason Snoopy had died on the day that he did was because of my work and my family and a lack of alternative ways to take care of his needs as an elderly dog at the end of his life. I had to accept all over again that Snoopy's euthanasia was not only about suffering, it was about practicality.

What was most surprising about this revelation was that rather than making me feel worse about the decision I had made, I finally felt better. Now that events out of my control had enabled me to review my decision, I finally accepted that letting Snoopy go because I could not care *for* him at that time, did not mean that I cared *about* him any less. Of course, this does not sound especially radical logic, or even new to the veterinary euthanasia debate, but what struck me was how powerful this idea of separating caring *for* and caring *about* Snoopy was for me emotionally.

Throughout my career as a veterinary surgeon I have been exposed to the argument that euthanasia is in the best interests of animals who are suffering. This professional focus on the wellbeing of the animal patient might easily be translated into the 'caring for' element of veterinary end-of-life decision-making, where euthanasia may be framed as a caring intervention which aims to alleviate animal patients' suffering. What my long career did not prepare me for was the emotional consequences of euthanasia involving an animal I cared *about*. Indeed, I believe that the euthanasia of my own pet was made more difficult by my unpreparedness in this regard; I expected to feel that I had done the right thing. I had been involved in countless euthanasia procedures as a veterinary professional and many had been incredibly sad and upsetting. The guilt and regret I felt after the euthanasia of my own pet, however, was unlike anything I had experienced before.

My experiences of guilt and grief are all too commonly reported, with decision-making regarding companion animal euthanasia reportedly both intensifying grief and resulting in potentially long lasting feelings of guilt and failure (Morris, 2012). Even where pet owners feel that euthanasia is the humane option, it has been shown that approximately half of pet owners report retrospective questioning of their decision and feelings of guilt (Adams et al, 2000). Here I want to propose that tension between our practical (caring for) and emotional (caring about) relationships with pets creates an environment where pet owners must logically request euthanasia to avoid inevitable suffering, yet at the same time their emotional attachments compel them to nurture and to preserve life, preventing an emotional acceptance of euthanasia as the correct course of action.

Here I want to pause for a moment to briefly highlight the role that my many identities have undoubtedly played in *diffracting* (Barad, 2007) the multiple angles and aspects of end-of-life care that this chapter explores. In this chapter I have been a pet owner so far, but in this section my argument is further developed through my role as a veterinary surgeon and the identification of tensions between my experiences of euthanasia from these different perspectives. Next I will become a relative and a carer, while throughout I am unashamedly a researcher, a scholar and an activist. Each of these lenses brings into focus the effects of differences in the meaning of care and experiences at the end of a life. My aim is to demonstrate the value of thinking *across* these effects, to expose the positive consequences of alternative perspectives within a specific debate.

In later sections I explore the implications of tensions between caring for and caring about animals for end-of-life care practices. First I show how this knowledge, gained through my experiences with Snoopy, also helped me to deal with the loss of a human family member. I aim to demonstrate how conceptual knowledge such as this might usefully be extended *across* the care of humans and non-human animals.

Dementia, guilt and grief

Later that summer something else significant changed for me as a close family member was admitted to a care home with advanced dementia. She spent the last few weeks of her life there, with family and friends unable to visit her due to COVID-19 restrictions. This situation was not unique to our family, there are widespread accounts of the radical changes which were imposed on how and where end-of-life care was provided for both humans and animals. The social distancing requirements and hospital and care home visiting restrictions in 2020 drastically and unbearably changed the nature of relationships between the dying and all those who loved them.

I was able to see my relative once before she passed away, she was recovering from a recent fall and was seated in a wheelchair with a nasty bruise on her face. The care assistant pushed the chair up to a glass door which was opened a crack to allow me to speak to her from outside, where I stood in my coat in a heavy summer downpour. My relative did not look like herself, she was pale and thin and seemed shrunken as she sat huddled in the chair under a blanket. 'Look who has come to see you!' exclaimed the care assistant as she leaned over the chair to point me out through the glass. 'It's Vanessa!' The silver-haired bruised head jerked up from its drooping position 'Ness?' her weak voice tremored, and I flinched at the sound of her pet name for me. 'Yes it's me' I nodded. Her face lit up with the biggest smile and as her milky eyes locked onto mine I felt the most extraordinary sensation, a rushing feeling with such an intensity it was as if some nameless, invisible energy was passing between us. I could almost hear it crackling. It was familiarity, it was recognition, it was memory, love, hope and desperation all communicated in a fraction of a second.

'How lovely to see you' she exclaimed politely, her eyes glued to my face as this intense wordless data transfer also continued. It felt as if the everyday language was a front to disguise the real message that was passing between us. 'Do come in, how was your journey down and where are the children? Are you going to stay for lunch?' It was clear that our conversation was, in her mind, taking place several years previously when I used to visit her at her house with my children. The words that she said to me felt just as if we were really there, but her eyes were not saying the same thing. My own voice felt compelled to go there too and I apologised that I had not brought the children and that I could not come in or stay for lunch but that I had just wanted to see her. A growing lump in my throat threatened to derail me as she made it clear that she was disappointed and made me promise to stay for longer next time I was passing. 'I must go now', I finally blurted, and as she looked away from me, confused, the breaking of that intense and wordless bond between us was almost unbearable. 'Are you going too?' she asked the care assistant, twisting round to look up at her face like a frightened child. 'No I'm not going anywhere' came the laughing reply as the care assistant stroked her hair away from her bruised face, 'I'm always here'. I left them to it and walked away from the closed glass door with my tears joining the raindrops coursing down my face.

I was not allowed to visit again. As her health continued to deteriorate I was in contact with the care home almost daily and they patiently described what she had eaten, how she was feeling and what I could send to make her feel more comfortable. I felt desperate to see her, but I remember being able to choose a pair of slippers for her online from the Marks and Spencer's website and it feeling like the most important and significant decision that I was ever going to make. I can still remember poring anxiously over the multiple pages of different options and the joy and relief of hearing over the telephone that they fitted her and that she was walking a few steps in them.

When she died at the end of the summer my feelings of grief and guilt returned like familiar friends. My brain and body knew just how to respond to this situation and I quickly slipped into a pattern of mourning that already felt well practised. It felt so familiar to be questioning what might have changed had I been able to do more for her. To be asking how I could ever forgive myself for abandoning her at her time of need and for leaving her alone when I should have been eating with her, talking to her and holding her hand. Yet again, the logical side of me knew that I had had no choice, but it could not prevent my emotional side from attacking me. It was the rehearsal for this moment that I had been a part of when Snoopy died which saved me from myself in the end.

I spent time thinking about the new understanding I had reached after processing my feelings about Snoopy's death. I realised that the same explanation fitted my current situation perfectly. I knew that I had not been able to care *for* my relative in the way that I wanted to, but I reminded myself that this did not mean that I had not cared *about* her as much as I should have done. Whatever may be said about family relationships and the place of animals within them, I must report that for me these situations felt almost identical, emotionally at least. Just as my body and mind had recognised the previous feelings of grief and guilt which had resurfaced again at this time, so too where they able to recognise the comfort that this new understanding had brought. Again I was able to recognise that I did not need to feel guilty for practical failures which were out of my control, and that I had still loved her as much as I should have done.

What is important about this story is a recognition of cross-species learning in understanding and practising end-of-life 'care'. My experiences of loss and grief after family bereavement were changed because of the loss of Snoopy and what I had learnt from that. While this may not seem like a momentous discovery on a personal level, it throws into relief the lack of formal communication which currently exists across disciplines, professions and species when it comes to studying, planning and practising end-of-life care. What might it mean for these fields if we acknowledged, embraced or even positively encouraged cross-species learning of the type that I have described?

Veterinary euthanasia, personhood and care

In this volume, the pathophysiological similarities between human and non-human animals, especially mammals, are highlighted through shared experiences of dementia and related neurodegenerative disorders. While some animals experience neurodegenerative disease as models for human health research, others experience naturally occurring disease, such as canine cognitive dysfunction (CCD) which is fairly commonly diagnosed in elderly pet dogs (Osella et al, 2007). While veterinary medical treatment is believed to be beneficial in managing the symptoms of this disease, pet owners are also advised to make lifestyle changes to help their dog cope better with their symptoms. Pet owners are advised to take their dog out for toileting more often, to rearrange their furniture, to spend more quality time with their dog and to use a pet sitter if they need to be left for a period of time (Vets4Pets, nd). The point I wish to make here is that the owners of dogs with CCD may be very likely to find, as I did with Snoopy, that they are unable to care *for* their dog because of these extra demands, however much they care *about* them.

While our society accepts the killing of animals for a variety of reasons, it is the place of the pet as a family member which makes the decision to end their life on practical grounds so difficult to bear. Classic ethnographic scholarship on the topic of veterinary euthanasia (Sanders, 1995: 211) conceptualises pet animals as both persons and non-persons, whereby they may be both loved, grieved *and* disposed of conveniently in the veterinary clinic. Sanders (1995) argues that 'It is here in the contested realm between persons and non-persons that we may gain significant insight into social relationships and the emotional experiences generated as these experiences are interactionally played out or ultimately terminated'. A clear point of interest here is the identification of a realm between personhood and non-personhood being claimed on behalf of pet animals, but which may also be experienced and explored in different ways by and for people living with dementia. It is in this space, we are told, that we may gain significant insight into social relationships and emotional experiences. I suggest here that these insights may not necessarily be limited in the scope of their application by species.

Returning to pets, I suggest that their liminal position on the fringes of personhood is even more complex when viewed through the lens of care. While we may care *about* our pets in very similar ways to other family members, we cannot usually care *for* them in the same ways, especially when they reach the end of their lives. What it means to care *about* an animal as a family member is therefore emotionally in tension with the challenges associated with caring *for* a pet at the end of their life. In a contemporary family setting there is no social care support for animals, no paid leave or benefits for animal carers, and I believe that it is this structural or practical distinction between human and animal end-of-life care provision which both justifies and necessitates the euthanasia of most pet animals.

It is our (in)capacity to care *for* appropriately which is the most powerful tool in separating accepted end-of-life approaches for humans and non-human family members. This argument is perhaps supported by the recent emergence of palliative and hospice care provision for pets, although there is little consensus within the veterinary profession regarding the appropriateness of euthanasia or palliative care as end-of-life treatments for animals (Kipperman et al, 2018; Dickinson and Hoffmann, 2019). As such it may be argued that efforts to develop an alternative route to caring *for* pets at the end of their lives, through extending human palliative care practices towards animals, troubles accepted ideas of morality and personhood in the veterinary clinic. For example, addressing the necessity of and justifications for pet animal euthanasia poses potentially bigger questions should it become linked to critical thinking regarding the fate of other animals under veterinary care.

These concepts of caring *for* and caring *about* thus both shape and separate the contemporary landscapes in veterinary and medical understandings of end-of-life 'care'. I have shown how my shared experiences of caring for and about both human and non-human family members have allowed me to broaden my understanding of the meaning of care at the end of a life. I have also suggested that recognising the implications of caring *for* and caring *about* non-human family members is essential in veterinary end-of-life care and that this distinction may play a key role in understanding the grief and guilt associated with companion animal euthanasia.

In the final section, I broaden my thinking further towards more theoretical and conceptual ideas of care and interspecies entanglements and argue for their place in realising future visions of end-of-life care.

Interspecies entanglements and speculative end-of-life 'care'

In this volume we finally give voice to the multitude of ways that humans and non-human animals are connected through chronic neurodegenerative disease. In this chapter I have so far shared some personal experiences of the ways that the end-of-life care of human and non-human animal family members may be experienced as both alike and distinct, including in the case of dementia-related illness, and what we may learn from this. I have used the unique backdrop of the COVID-19 pandemic to highlight the tensions which exist between caring for and caring about family members of any species at the end of their lives and the clinical implications of separating these concepts for our practices of care across species. I end now with thoughts on the relevance of cross-species thinking for embedding speculative, conceptual and theoretical approaches to care in everyday end-of-life care practices.

In end-of-life care practices, thinking across species boundaries may help us to make more far-reaching progress towards better outcomes for all. For example, in human patients, informal care provision in the family home has been contemplated in terms of the potential welfare impacts of caring *for* and caring *about* family members. It is suggested that both forms of care may impact upon the welfare of those supporting (human) patients, with the proposal that both 'caregiving' and 'family' welfare effects are considered in healthcare economies (Bobinac et al, 2010). In professional care home nursing, the replacement of protective modes of caring *for* patients with an increased focus on remedial models of caring *about* patients has been proposed, with the aim of promoting patient self-help and autonomy (Wild et al, 2012).

However, comparable work in the form of exploring the impacts of each type of care for pet owners and veterinary staff, and the potential to further reshape our approaches to end-of-life care beyond the development of practical or protective modes have yet to be explored in the context of non-human family members. This is just one example of the potential practical value of thinking *across* the end-of-life care of both human and non-human species.

Yet practical change does not always need to begin with end-of-life care practices. In this chapter I have used my experiences in end-of-life care to draw together knowledge from different settings. However, there is a growing body of work which explores the complexity of interrelations between humans and non-human animals from an overarching theoretical perspective and which may inform our interactions with one another across any and all settings. For example, the term interspecies entanglement encapsulates a theoretical perspective which views human and non-human animal relations though multiple, complex, untidy and ever-changing connections and disconnections (Latimer, 2013; Haraway, 2016). Lori Gruen (2015) applies such thinking to argue that our entangled relationships require us to extend empathy between species. Entangled empathy, it is argued, is a universal ethical approach which requires us to emotionally evaluate another's position, regardless of their species, in order to determine what, if anything, we are called upon to do (Gruen, 2015). We have seen in this chapter some of the ways that such an approach may allow us to better understand specific aspects of end-of-life care across species, but what might we learn from starting our explorations through such a theoretical lens? Where might our understanding of chronic neurodegenerative disease and end-of-life care take us if we applied such thinking routinely?

As a further example of how a different theoretical standpoint might alter future developments in end-of-life care, in my own recent work I have proposed that engagement with feminist care approaches may help us to develop our understanding of the complex realities of practising veterinary medicine (Ashall, 2022). I suggest that emotional, contextual and material experiences in the veterinary clinic are rarely explored for their significance in veterinary decision-making and that the impacts of veterinary interventions on animals, owners, staff and society are thus poorly understood.

These alternative theoretical lenses, which expose alternative perspectives on interspecies relationships and highlight the role of emotions, might require us to ask different questions about the future of end-of-life care. From the experiences I have shared in this chapter we might be permitted to ask: What is the significance of the emotions we experience when caring for and about animals, for the future of end-of-life care? Why is it so difficult to separate our emotional responses to caring *about* an individual from our practical desire to care *for* them? What is the significance of the natural desire to care *for* those whom we care *about*?

Martin et al (2015: 625) describe care as a 'slippery' concept. While we are all accustomed to this word, its precise meaning is often unclear and how it is used in one setting can be contradictory to its use elsewhere, as I have aimed to demonstrate here. Developing multi-species approaches to dementia studies will thus entail embracing the complexity and contradiction of care as a concept to be applied across species. For example, Martin et al suggest that:

> The very concept of care is not only multifaceted and contextual, but also suggests different political commitments, inspiring a range of different ethics and forms of intervention. This is part of care's

> productivity. For this reason, there can be no singular vision of what care is or what it might become. (Martin et al, 2015: 634)

In terms of what care might become and what it might achieve in multi-species dementia studies, Puig de la Bellacasa (2017: 5) describes three dimensions of care – labour, emotion and politics – and argues that the unsolved tensions and relations between these dimensions are in themselves a meaningful terrain for exploring 'how to care' in more-than-human worlds. This speculative work points us towards a radical rethinking of what care means, brought about through broadening our concept of the world beyond the human. Might we argue then that through broadening our concept of dementia beyond the human, we may also develop our ideas of what dementia 'care' is and could be?

In closing, my own experiences of caring for both humans and non-humans at the end of life have shown me how challenging it can be to deal with imbalances between emotional and practical aspects of care, but also how useful it is to identify and separate these concepts. I have aimed to show that speculative and conceptual work in human–animal relationships and concepts of care requires us to embrace this complexity and to contemplate where we may need to make changes to our existing practices. Giraud (2019) reminds us that recognition of interspecies entanglements is not sufficient, in itself, to ensure good outcomes for all those involved. As such, engagement with conceptual and speculative approaches to caring human–animal relations should be contemplated for their value in developing practical proposals for the future of end-of-life care. In this way, we may strive to make end-of-life care across species, including for those who are living with neurodegenerative disease, a place where caring becomes the foundational reason behind practical change.

References

Adams, C.L., Bonnet, B.N. and Meek, A.H. (2000) 'Predictors of owner response to companion animal death in 177 clients from 14 practices in Ontario', *J Am Vet Med Assoc*, 217(9): 1303–1309.

Adams, T.E., Holman Jones, S. and Ellis, C. (eds) (2016) *Handbook of Autoethnography*, New York, NY: Routledge.

Ashall, V. (2022) 'A feminist ethic of care for the veterinary profession', *Frontiers in Veterinary Science*, 9: 795628.

Barad, K. (2007) *Meeting the Universe Halfway*, Durham, NC: Duke University Press.

Bobinac, A., Job, N., Van Exel, A., Rutten, F., Werner, F.H. and Brouwer, B.F. (2010) 'Caring for and caring about: Disentangling the caregiver effect and the family effect', *Journal of Health Economics*, 29(4): 549–556.

Dickinson, G. and Hoffmann, H.C. (2019) 'Animal hospice and palliative care: Veterinarians' experiences and preferred practices', *Journal of Veterinary Behavior*, 32: 57–61.

Giraud, E.H. (2019) *What Comes After Entanglement?*, Durham, NC: Duke University Press.

Gruen, L. (2015) *Entangled Empathy: An Alternative Ethic for Our Relations with Animals*, Brooklyn, NY: Lantern Books.

Haraway, D. (2016) *Staying With the Trouble: Making Kin in the Cthulucene*, Durham, NC: Duke University Press.

Kipperman, B., Morris, P. and Rollin, B. (2018) 'Ethical dilemmas encountered by small animal veterinarians: Characterisation, responses, consequences and beliefs regarding euthanasia', *Veterinary Record*, 182(19): 548.

Latimer, J. (2013) 'Being alongside: Rethinking relations amongst different kinds', *Theory, Culture & Society*, 30(7–8): 77–104.

Martin, A., Myers, N. and Viseu, A. (2015) 'The politics of care in technoscience', *Social Studies of Science*, 45(5): 625–641.

Morris, P.M. (2012) *Blue Juice: Euthanasia in Veterinary Medicine*, Philadelphia, PA: Temple University Press.

Osella, M.C., Re, G., Odore, R., Girardi, C., Badino, P., Barbero, R., et al (2007) 'Canine cognitive dysfunction syndrome: Prevalence, clinical signs and treatment with a neuroprotective nutraceutical', *Applied Animal Behaviour Science*, 105(4): 297–310.

Puig de la Bellacasa, M. (2017) *Matters of Care: Speculative Ethics in More Than Human Worlds*, Minneapolis, MN: University of Minnesota Press.

Sanders, C. (1995) 'Killing with kindness: Veterinary euthanasia and the social construction of personhood', *Sociological Forum*, 10: 195–214.

St. Pierre, E.A. (2021) Why post qualitative inquiry? *Qualitative Inquiry*, 27(2): 163–166.

Vets4Pets (nd) *Dementia in Dogs*. Available from: https://www.vets4pets.com/pet-health-advice/dog-advice/dementia-in-dogs/ [Accessed 30 November 2022].

Wild, D., Nelson, S., Szczepura, A. and Kydd, A. (2012) 'Caring for and caring about 1: A new model of care for the older person', *Nursing Times*, 108(12): 12–14.

7

Personhood and dementia: a multi-species view

Nicholas Jenkins, Anna Jack-Waugh and Louise Ritchie (with Anne Rankin)

Introduction

Personhood and dementia are two concepts with an entangled history. Ever since the European Enlightenment (1685–1815), Western societies have conceptualised personhood in ways that construct an insuperable divide between human beings and all other species. The Enlightenment philosopher John Locke (1632–1704), for example, viewed a person as 'a thinking intelligent being that has reason and reflection and can consider itself as itself' (Locke, 1689, cited in Gordon-Roth, 2020). For Locke, our personhood stems from the exceptional ability of human beings to, among other things, create memories, exercise reason or rational judgement, and demonstrate self-awareness. It was within this philosophical tradition that dementia, as a distinct category of mental disorder, first emerged within psychiatric nosology during the late 18th century. Inspired by Locke's empiricist view of personhood, pioneers of modern psychiatry such as Philippe Pinel (1745–1826) and Jean-Etienne Esquirol (1772–1840) sought to define dementia, not as the absence of personhood, but as the corruption of those very faculties which Locke viewed as fundamental to it (see, for example, Pinel, 1806).

Despite their entangled histories, it was not until the latter decades of the 20th century that personhood re-emerged as a keystone concept within dementia studies. Allied to the rise of modern biomedicine in the early 20th century, and as Peel et al highlight in Chapter 5, commentators argued that dementia had become likened to a form of *social death*, within which the personhood of the 'sufferer' was gradually and irretrievably eroded by the progression of neurocognitive disorder (see, for example, Cohen and Eisdorfer, 1986; Sweeting and Gilhooly, 1997). Led by the work of Tom Kitwood and colleagues, the Personhood movement of the 1980s and 1990s sought fundamentally to challenge this way of thinking. It argued that the tendency within Western societies to equate personhood with the individual's capacity for agency, consciousness, reason and rationality served to dehumanise people with dementia and to position them outside of 'The Personhood Club' (Kitwood, 1997: 9). Drawing inspiration from the work of Martin Buber, Carl Rogers and Maurice Merleau-Ponty, Kitwood sought to recast our understandings of personhood in ways that were better suited to truly *seeing* the person living with dementia (see Kitwood, 1997; Kitwood and Bredin, 1992). For Kitwood, this involved a fundamental (ontological) shift. In his hands, personhood was no longer defined in relation to intrinsic cognitive abilities but, rather, via the world of social relations. From this perspective, humans become persons through their everyday interactions with other human beings. Personhood thus became something to be accomplished through everyday acts of care. This way of thinking led Kitwood (1997: 8) to his seminal definition of personhood, as 'a standing or status that is bestowed upon one human being, by others, in the context of relationship and social being'.

The rise of the Personhood movement had a profound impact upon the everyday worlds of dementia. It led to new, *person*-centred approaches to care and to new forms of care practice, most notably Dementia Care Mapping (for example, Bradford Dementia Group, 1997). While highly influential, the view of personhood advocated by Kitwood and colleagues has not been without its critics. Bartlett and O'Connor (2007; 2010), for example, argue that Kitwood's view of personhood overly focused attention on micro-social environments, especially the immediate care setting, and thus failed to consider sufficiently the socio-political contexts in which dementia is experienced. Adopting an intersectional lens, others such as Hulko (2004) continue this line of critique, arguing that established approaches do not sufficiently consider the ways in which discrimination in dementia crosses over with other systems of oppression such as gender, class and race. Writing from a practice-focused perspective, Nolan et al critique the development of person-centredness in health and social care, arguing that 'some have begun to doubt if person-centred care can actually be achieved, and to question whether it is simply an evangelical ideal' (Nolan et al, 2004: 46).

Although critiques of person-centred approaches to dementia are many and varied, what is rarely critiqued (or even questioned) is the continued reliance upon human exceptionalist and binary forms of thinking. While the Personhood movement may have broadened our understandings of what constitutes a person, champions of person-centred approaches nevertheless appear comfortable with the idea that *The Personhood Club* has an exclusive membership, and that membership should be extended to 'humans' alone. By continuing to adopt this way of thinking, person-centred practice risks reenforcing the implicit idea that personhood is both an exceptional (that is, mono-species) and morally superior (that is, discriminatory) form of Being. This is a way of thinking that has, over the centuries, come to position various populations – including women, Black people and disabled people, not to mention all animals – as outside of *The Personhood Club* to begin with (Wolfe, 2003; 2010; Braidotti, 2013).

Across the humanities and social sciences, there is growing recognition that we humans live in a multi-species world. This 'multispecies turn' (Reiger and Bolinski, 2020) is bringing increased recognition that humans are not ontologically distinct from all other Beings and that we exist as humans precisely because we exist within complex and entangled webs of multi-species relations. As the sociobiologist Richard O. Wilson (1993: 39) states: 'Humanity did not soft-land into the teeming biosphere, like an alien from another planet. We arose from other organisms already here, whose great diversity, conducting experiment upon experiment in the production of new life forms, eventually hit upon the human species.'

From a multi-species perspective, personhood is not an exclusively human affair. This – it is important to note – is separate from claims that members of other species should be granted legal personhood alongside human beings. Several compelling arguments have been made in favour of extending legal personhood to other sentient beings, such as gorillas, orangutans and other hominids, based on their capacity for 'human-like' thinking (see, for example, The Great Ape Project[1]). These, however, are separate from debates about what constitutes human personhood. From a multi-species perspective, the human condition is not ontologically distinct and set apart from the rest of existence, which is a view that has tended to dominate Western thinking since at least the writings of Rene Descartes (1637; 1641, reprinted, 1993). Rather, it holds that humans are made persons through their relations with other species and therefore cannot exist independently, as persons, outside of those relations. Further, it assumes that our relations with other species are both inter-active and *intra*-active (Barad, 2007; Haraway, 2008). They produce *Cuts* (Barad, 2007) in the socio-material world and these *Cuts*, in turn, create worldly distinctions upon which the foundations of personhood are built. This way of thinking, which often falls under the moniker of the *posthuman*, has much to offer dementia studies. With some notable exceptions (for example, DeFalco, 2016; Quinn and Blandon, 2017; 2020), posthumanism has yet to permeate the dementia debate or to inform dementia-related practice.

This chapter was inspired by a desire to explore how multi-species thinking might reinvigorate the personhood debate and create new opportunities for practising person-centredness in dementia. What follows is not a definitive multi-species theory of personhood, nor does it present the reader with an 'oven-ready' set of practices to be implemented within dementia settings. What we hope to initiate is a way of thinking about personhood and about person-centredness in dementia that can incorporate more than what the logic of human exceptionalism prescribes. Our discussion begins with the body and embodiment in dementia and how human bodies are made of more than human elements alone. We then consider relations with *Other* (animal) bodies and how these relations may be incorporated within person-centred approaches to dementia. From there, we advocate for the practising of *response-ability* that better recognises how people with dementia and animals each become with the other, within the everyday worlds of dementia.

Personhood, dementia and the (multi-species) body

Dementia is fundamentally an embodied experience as, to experience dementia, one must first experience a body. Since the early 2000s, researchers have paid close attention to the body and to the relationship between dementia, embodiment and personhood. Kontos (2005), for example, argues that the body is a primordial site within which personhood is expressed through pre-reflexive and spontaneous movement, which Kontos refers to as *embodied habitus*. Attending to embodied habitus, Kontos argues, provides insights into the personhood of the subject living with dementia long after the capacity for language or reflexive self-awareness may have been affected by neurocognitive disease. In a similar vein, Twigg argues that the presentation of the body through dress (Twigg, 2010) and inter-corporeal forms of 'bodywork' (Twigg et al, 2011) provide opportunities for the expression of embodied subjectivity within everyday dementia settings. Indeed, Kitwood himself argued that personhood is an embodied state of Being, as opposed to a metaphysical one. He suggested that interpersonal relations that promote and impede personhood leave material imprints that may manifest themselves upon the body, including the brain of the person with dementia (Kitwood, 1997).

Important as these early contributions have been in highlighting the centrality of the body in dementia, they all begin from the anthropocentric assumption that embodiment is an exclusively human affair, which it is not. Human bodies are complex landscapes of multi-species relations. Approximately 10 per cent of our deoxyribonucleic acid (DNA), for example, is non-human in origin having entered the human genome via endosymbiosis (Sagan, 1967) and other mechanisms associated with horizontal gene transfer (Crisp et al, 2015). Although estimates vary among microbiologists, it is generally accepted that most of the cells that make up human bodies are not human but are, instead, a rich milieu of protists, archaea, fungi, bacteria and viruses residing both on and under the skin (Gilbert et al, 2012). These microscopic 'critters' (Haraway, 2008) do not live passively within the body but actively shape the visceral landscapes they inhabit, forming complex microbiomes. Microbiomes are formed in the body before birth, in utero, and develop throughout the life course well into the third and fourth age. Biologically speaking, there is nothing mono-species about human bodies. Our bodies are dynamic, complex, multi-species *assemblages* that are accomplished through a myriad of microscopic, multi-species relationships.

Although biomedical research has yet to explore fully the scope and variety of our intra-corporeal relations with other species, it is becoming increasingly apparent that these critters play pivotal roles in shaping embodied experience. Indeed, changes within microbiomes over time are now thought to correlate with trajectories of human ageing, health, illness and disease (Bana and Cabreiro, 2019). As microbiologists Crilly et al argue in this volume (Chapter 4), there is already good scientific evidence to suggest long-term changes within microbiomes, which interact with processes of *inflammaging*, may correlate with the onset of Alzheimer's disease and other dementia-related conditions. Much of the current research is driven by a desire to develop new interventions for the prevention, treatment and management of dementia-related disease. Important as new interventions are, emergent understandings of bodies as multi-species accomplishments point to new ways of understanding personhood. As Haraway (2008; 2016) argues, what is on offer here is an alternative to the dominant Western metanarratives, which have tended to equate personhood with the body's capacity for autonomy, individuality and to exist in autopoiesis. Such narratives, Haraway argues, maintain the idea of an insuperable divide between Self and Other, and between what is human and what is not. What emerges in its stead is an understanding of embodied subjectivity as always accomplished in *sympoesis* (making with) (Haraway, 2016). Thus, Haraway (2008: 1) argues, 'I become an adult being in company with these tiny messmates'. There are, in other words, no neat divides between human and non-human, the person and the (non)person. Embodied subjectivity is never discrete nor static but always changing and always made with other species. In the words of biologists Gilbert et al (2012), we humans have never been 'individuals', if to Be an individual is to Be an autonomous (mono-species) self. What we humans are, they argue, are holobionts. That is, 'integrated organism[s] comprised of both host elements and persistent populations of symbionts' (Gilbert et al, 2012: 237–238).

This reframing of embodied personhood has profound implications when thinking about person-centredness in dementia. According to Shildrick (2021) it *queers* our very understandings of what dementia is and of what dementia affects. Queer, in this context, is not used by Shildrick to refer to LGBTQIA+ individuals and communities. Rather, it is used as a verb, highlighting the radical potential of new ways of thinking. For Shildrick, contemporary approaches to dementia remain wedded to the idea that it signals a progressive and inevitable decline in the body's capacity to maintain both its independence and, ultimately, its inner subjectivity. From this assumption, the goal of much care practice has been to maintain or preserve the Self in the presence of dementia, for as long as possible. A multi-species understanding of embodied subjectivity *queers* this agenda, following Shildrick, because it rejects the very notion of a *Sovereign Self* that resides within the body and comes under attack from dementia. Rather, it reaches into the posthuman, by placing an emphasis on *zōē* as life existing within and beyond the ecology of the human body (see Braidotti, 2013). Because of this, Shildrick argues, *flourishing* becomes possible well into the advanced stages of dementia and, indeed, even beyond the death of the body itself. This is because death of the body does not signify the end of Being, but a transformation of biological matter in ways that give rise to new possibilities of life's becoming. To embrace flourishing, therefore, involves:

> [E]mbracing uncertainty and radical change, and sustaining becoming, however that plays out, even in the face of disease, disability, dementia, and impending death. Flourishing does not simply refer to the conditions of living, but has a wider meaning in which the event of death enables life itself to recompose under new relations of sustainability. (Shildrick, 2021: 95–96)

Shildrick's posthuman ethic of flourishing aligns closely with non-Western, Buddhist ontology. The concept of Inter-Being, for example, first proposed by the exiled Vietnamese monk Thich Nhat Hanh (1991; 2017), highlights how no body exists in isolation, and that each body is always connected to all other bodies through complex webs of relations. As such, Thich Nhat Hanh argues, we humans always *Inter-Are* with all other forms of life. To practice an ethic of flourishing is to resist the urge to cling to a social representation of an individual self and instead, to embrace the fluidity, interconnectedness, and the perpetual impermanence of embodied personhood. Personhood – from this perspective – is valued precisely because it is the expression of something much greater than itself, namely *zōē*. We shall revisit the implications of this way of thinking in the final section of this chapter, but we believe, although contentious, it has potential to profoundly affect the everyday landscapes of dementia. At this point, however, we turn to relations between human and animal bodies, in inter-corporeal space, and consider how these too may form part of a person-centred approach to dementia.

Exploring the 'zoological dimension'

In his presidential address to the Southern Sociological Society, Clifton Bryant (1979) chastised sociologists around the world for failing to attend to the 'zoological dimension'. The social world, Bryant argues, is not composed of humans alone and animals have discernible impacts in virtually all aspects of social life. Thus, Bryant argues, researchers 'can no more appropriately ignore the zoological dimension, than an analysis of drama can ignore the seminal actors in a play' (Bryant, 1979: 417). It is abundantly clear that the everyday worlds of dementia are not composed of humans alone. From the laboratory to the care home, animals are on the scene, yet dementia studies and ageing studies have largely failed to attend to the zoological dimension or, for that matter, to grant animals any systematic attention at all. The rise of animal-assisted interventions and green care initiatives, such as care farming and forest bathing, however, are bringing the more-than-human world into sharper relief. While researchers appear willing to explore the therapeutic effects that may arise from people with dementia interacting with animals (for example, Yakimicki et al, 2019) or immersing in nature (for example, Evans et al, 2019), what remains under-researched and under-theorised are the ways in which these may be considered part of the social accomplishment of personhood.

Failure to consider the role of more-than-human actors in the social accomplishment of personhood appears to stem more from anthropocentric ideology than from any robust evidence to suggest other bodies do not matter. According to Merleau-Ponty (1968), inter-corporeality (the sharing of embodied experience) stems from the body's existential status as a *chiasm*; a crossing-over of objective and subjective worlds, which, by enfolding these worlds within itself, makes both objective and subjective realities possible. Our *sensibility*, Merleau-Ponty argues, does not stem from our transcendental belonging to some uniquely and exclusively human form of consciousness, as the philosopher Edmund Husserl (1859–1938) believed. Rather, according to Merleau-Ponty, it stems from the participatory relationship that exists between subject and object, the sentient and the sensed. Although Merleau-Ponty died before fully articulating his understanding of inter-corporeality, we have yet to find any indication in his writings that he considered it to be exclusive to human bodies. Indeed, we find it interesting that at key points in his work, Merleau-Ponty refers to 'organisms', rather than humans, when discussing the importance of inter-corporeality. For example:

> Why would not the synergy exist among different *organisms*, if it is possible within each? Their landscapes interweave, their actions and their passions fit together exactly: this is possible as soon as we no longer make belongingness to one same 'consciousness' the primordial definition of sensibility, and as soon as we rather understand it as the return of the visible upon itself, a carnal adherence of the sentient to the sensed and of the sensed to the sentient. (Merleau-Ponty, 1968: 142; italics added)

If we reject the Cartesian notion that animal bodies are biological automata, inherently incapable of subjective experience, and we assume instead that animal bodies like human bodies possess the potential for inter-corporeality, it follows that the interactions between human bodies and animal bodies contain more than the potential for the former to take pleasure from the latter. Rather, it follows that what may be present within these embodied interactions is a sharing of subjective experience; a mutual and *trans-species Being-in-the-world* (Wolfe, 2010). If we apply this way of thinking to the interactions that take place within, for example, animal assisted therapies and other forms of human–animal interaction, we create opportunities to view these interactions in a different light. They become visible as person-generating and relationship-generating forms of inter-corporeal exchange.

Research suggests members of neuro-diverse communities may relate to animals in ways that may not be replicated when interacting with humans (for example, Malcolm et al, 2018). Practitioners have previously observed how people with dementia who otherwise appear withdrawn and noncommunicative may 'come alive' in the presence of animals (for example, Care Inspectorate, 2018). Multi-species interaction may be rich sites for inter-corporeality in dementia, yet we lack the conceptual toolkit to explore these sufficiently. We know, however, that like many other holobionts, human bodies possess deep-seated, pre-reflexive tendencies for responding to non-human animals, and that these tendencies are species-specific. Encounters with exotic birds, horses and companion dogs, for example, tend to evoke different visceral responses to those experienced when encountering snakes, spiders or other reptilian predators. These pre-reflexive tendencies, as Kellert (1993) observes, are remarkably consistent across human societies and cultures. Several concepts have been articulated to explain these tendencies, including *biophilia* (Wilson, 1984), *biophobia* (Ulrich, 1993) and the *human–animal bond*. Following Sagan and Margulis (1993), we prefer the notion of *prototaxis*. First articulated by evolutionary biologist Ivan E. Wallin, prototaxis refers to the 'tendency of one organism or cell to react in a definite manner to another organism or cell' (Wallin, 1923, cited in Sagan and Margulis, 1993: 346). Unlike biophilia or the human–animal bond, prototaxis is rooted in the observable behaviour of bodies as opposed to abstract notions of joy, fear or awe. This makes prototaxis useful on two fronts. First, it is a less anthropocentric concept as it relates to the behaviours of human and more-than-human bodies. This enables us to explore prototaxis within bodies (for example, as the interaction of microscopic organisms) as well as between bodies as the interaction of humans and other animals. Second, prototaxis does not assume that visceral responses are inherent or that all members of the same species possess the same deep-seated capacity for response. Lived experience and embodied memories are likely to be key factors affecting each body's prototaxis, in addition to any genetic predispositions that might be present. In this respect, we can think of prototaxis as a multi-species companion concept to Kontos' notion of the embodied habitus. In other words, as 'the primordial capacity of the body to pre-reflectively perform' (Kontos, 2005: 560) when encountering members of other species.

Following Abrams (1996), encounters involving people with dementia and animals may evoke the body's pre-reflexive capacity for *synesthesia.* Within medical lexicon, synesthesia typically refers to a pathological state of perception, in which sense data become conflated, such as when people report 'smelling' colours or 'tasting' sounds. In Abram's diction, however, it refers to an intense and lively state of bodily awareness, in which the senses of the body are engaged as 'a single, hyperattentive organ' such as when 'we feel ourselves listening with our eyes and watching with our ears, ready to respond with our whole body to any change in the Other's behaviour' (Abrams, 1996: 130). Encounters involving humans and animals, Abrams argues, often engage the body's pre-reflexive capacity for synesthetic experience. The reasons for this, he argues, are likely to be evolutionary in origin as, for thousands of years, humans have relied upon their abilities to tune in with the entirety of their bodies to the presence of other species, such as when hunting or when fleeing from predators. While such capacities are no longer required for physical survival they remain, Abrams argues, deeply rooted within the bodies of humans and other animals. However, not all humans (including people affected by dementia) respond positively to the presence of other animals. One explanation for this, as the founding father of animal assisted therapy Boris Levinson (1907–1984) highlights, is that while animals have occupied central roles within human societies for thousands of years – and the human body has changed little in evolutionary terms over the past million years – the advent of our technologically driven societies has led to profound changes in how humans regard members of other species and engage with the 'natural' world. As Levinson (1972: 6) argues: 'As a result of our technological orientation, we see nature as a gigantic, inexhaustible mine of riches or, more destructively, as a whore to be exploited at leisure and then cast out.'

Estrangement from the more-than-human world is a key feature of late-capitalist societies and thus manifests itself within the everyday worlds of dementia. According to Abrams, its origins can be traced to the introduction of the phonetic alphabet in 400 BC, as this replaced idiographic writing systems based on representations of animals, plants and other elements of the more-than-human world, with abstract signs and symbols. This, he argues, served to decouple language from its carnal, animistic roots. With this, Abrams (1996) argues, came a new and profoundly inner sense of the Self as a form of subjectivity that is set apart from all other species. It is this sense of the Self that has come to dominate thinking about personhood in dementia for the past 200 years.

Towards response-ability in dementia

So far, we have explored embodiment (in dementia) as a multi-species accomplishment and inter-corporeality (in dementia) as a multi-species phenomenon. We draw on these two arguments in this final section, to apply the concept of response-ability as a framework for understanding what is truly 'at stake' (Haraway, 2008) when humans and other animals encounter each other within the everyday worlds of dementia.

Rooted in a feminist ethic of care (Tronto, 1993) and first developed by writers such as Haraway (2008; 2016) and Barad (2007), response-ability refers to the capacity of sentient bodies to be rendered capable of response (Bozalek and Zembylas, 2023). The capacity for response, to affect and become affected by the other, as Donna Haraway argues, is not an abstract quality nor one pre-determined by biology, but socially situated and specific to the ways in which bodies encounter each other within everyday worlds. In this respect, response-ability is qualitatively different to the concept of responsibility, which has its origins in an ethic of justice (Tronto, 1993). To practice responsibility is to be held accountable for one's actions and their consequences. To practice response-ability, as Haraway (2008: 19) argues, is: 'To hold in regard, to respond, to look back reciprocally, to notice, to pay attention, to have courteous regard for, to esteem: all of that is tied to polite greeting, to constituting the polis, where and when species meet.'

To practice response-ability, Haraway argues, is to work with others (both human and more-than-human) in the cultivation of the worlds we wish to live and die in. This, Haraway argues, is a difficult process as we must continue to inherit each other's histories and learn how to get along with each other in conditions where the outcomes are far from certain and where 'success' is not guaranteed. Following Haraway, becoming in dementia is a world-making process in which entanglements of humans and animals are knotted and re-knotted in complex ways. Thus, by becoming with each other within shared conditions of response-ability, people affected by dementia and animals have the potential to form new relations which, in turn, give rise to new possibilities for becoming.

The bodies of animals and humans encounter each other daily within the everyday worlds of dementia, yet many such encounters go unacknowledged. In care settings, for example, the bodies of animals are regularly consumed by people with dementia as a source of food. Before this encounter can occur, animal bodies must first be killed and rendered incapable of response, ensuring their transformation from sentient body-subjects into 'meat'. There is no mutual response-ability within such encounters. In contrast, when animal *Others* are regarded as minded companions, collaborators, co-inquisitors and co-investigators within the everyday worlds of dementia, conditions exist for new possibilities of becoming. As such, and following

Haraway, much is 'at stake' when people with dementia and animals meet each other within the everyday worlds of dementia. Personhood, mindedness and animality, we argue, are all at stake when species meet in dementia and the outcomes are far from assured.

We have already discussed the tendency within Western societies to equate personhood with the capacity for language, reason, reflection, agency, autonomy and self-awareness. This has historically positioned those living with dementia as *Other* to the liberal humanist ideal of personhood. Also, within Western societies, animals have tended not to be regarded as minded beings and, in consequence, not considered persons and thus not accorded the moral and legal privileges that the status of personhood confers. Working within the symbolic interactionist tradition, Gubrium (1986), Sabat and Harré (1992) and Kitwood (1997) were some of the first to highlight how mindedness in dementia is a social relationship and one that is not determined by biology alone. How paid carers and significant others interact with people with dementia, they argued, may facilitate as well as impede the social recognition of the person with dementia as a minded being worthy of dignity and respect. Drawing on this work, Arluke and Sanders (1996) similarly argued that mindedness in the context of human–animal interaction is a sociogenic feature of identity. How humans interact with each other and with animal *Others* can enable social recognition of the animal as a sentient and minded social actor. Mindedness, in other words, whether it is applied to human or more-than-human bodies, is a product of social relationships. By becoming minded, both human and animal bodies become response-able in the creation of everyday worlds. It is to this potential that our sense of response-ability refers. To illustrate this point, we draw upon the cultivation of response-ability within the Dementia Dog project in Scotland, UK.[2]

Established in Scotland, UK, in 2011, Dementia Dog is a collaboration between Alzheimer Scotland, the Glasgow School of Art and Dogs for Good. Initially centred around training dogs to assist people with dementia and placing them with couples on an indefinite basis, the project now provides a blueprint for a range of canine-assisted interventions across the world. As researchers, we have been involved with the project since 2016. We conducted a realist evaluation of the pilot phase (Ritchie et al, 2021) and developed a series of analytic vignettes to explore relations between dogs, carers and people with a diagnosis of dementia (Jenkins et al, 2021). Through our involvement with the project, we have been able to observe how the creation of multi-species caring triads led to unpredictable ways of becoming in the presence of dementia. We observed, for example, how becoming response-able within multi-species triads meant having to learn what was expected from the other, as well as adapting to the difficult, tumultuous and uncertain circumstances that are so often characteristic of the dementia journey. For some multi-species triads, it was a difficult experience and could affect the response-ability of the person with dementia and the dog in deleterious ways. For others, it generated new and enriching opportunities for becoming and for deep, personhood-generating forms of response-ability to emerge across species boundaries (Jenkins et al, 2021).

In the development of this chapter, we spoke with one carer, Anne, about her experiences of becoming with Uno. Uno is a bespoke trained Dementia Dog, who came to live with her and her husband, Henry, who Anne has known since she was 15 years old. Henry was diagnosed with vascular dementia several years ago and lived with the condition until his death in February 2022. As Anne told us, she and Henry were not a 'doggy family', before they were joined by Uno:

> We weren't a doggy family as such, but that changed when he [Uno] came. We certainly became a doggy family then, you know. He just fitted in, just as soon as we saw him, we knew he was the dog for us, and he accepted us very quickly as well. So he just became another member of the family.

Anne's recollections highlight how, by learning how to live together, and learning how to inherit each other's histories, a mutual, beyond words inter-corporeality developed between Uno and Henry. This enabled Uno to sense and respond to subtle changes in Henry's body; changes which were often imperceptible to Anne:

> So, from the get-go, the simplest things like … if Henry's blood sugar was low. He [Uno] sensed that before I did, and I didn't see, so that prevented hypos and things like that … he wasn't trained for that, he just knew. He would bark at Henry as though he says there's something wrong here, you know, and whether it was the smell of the acetone or whatever, the sweet smell they get. I don't know how he could sense it, but he would just bark and then sat down beside him and not move until I got the treatment.

This inter-corporeality, Anne further explained, extended beyond Uno's capacity to respond to changes in Henry's physiological state. It included an awareness and a capacity to respond to Henry's affective state as well:

> [H]e [Uno] knew when his [Henry's] mood was low. He knew when he was agitated. So it was, it was some situations were quite difficult until we got Uno and he regained himself. Sometimes he wouldn't even go out and you know, he would look out and say no, I'm not going out today because I don't want to. And Uno help[ed] with that as well. … He was a calming influence on him or I don't know why, but

> he didn't get agitated. Because he was always patting him. You know, he was always around, Uno was always at his feet. Always at his feet.

What Anne also showed us was how Henry's independence was very much 'at stake' within their dementia journey: '[Before Uno] [t]hings would have gone faster because I think Henry was beginning to kind of give up. What he thought he lost was his independence and you know how important his independence was to him.' With the addition of Uno to the caring assemblage, Anne described to us how Henry's independence was accomplished through the mutual interdependence that developed, over time, between Henry, Anne and Uno. In Anne's words, 'it became the triangle of care with Uno at the top and Henry and I both either side'. Henry, Anne and Uno developed a mutual propensity to affect and become affected by each other, in various and unpredictable ways. As Anne says, Uno could militate against some of the strains that developed within everyday life, such as when she and Henry would move at different 'paces': 'He [Henry] would think I would be nagging him. But you know, Uno doesn't nag. He [Henry] would sometimes get annoyed with me because I was either too slow or too fast. He used to say I do things too fast, that Uno does it at his pace.'

When outside and in social settings, the presence of Uno within the caring triad could enable the social accomplishment of Henry as a competent and minded social actor:

> [O]ne day we were in Sainsbury's and I was pushing the wheelchair and they people would come up and talk to Uno. But now if they go to Uno … they also talked to Henry. He kept social, you know, social circumstances, you know, they were conversations about Uno, but it was making Henry talk. … He used to boast about, you know, how good he [Uno] was and what he [Uno] did. And people were amazed … it was like a father and son relationship.

Anne also shared with us her grief of Henry dying, and about her sense of 'being one of two halves'. In this context, Anne also shared with us her love for Uno and the ways in which they are now united in their mutual grief for the loss of Henry:

> I really don't know how to describe what Uno does for me. He's just the light, you know, he's a light in my world. He just knows and he just comes over and just says, 'Mummy, I'll give you a cuddle and then you'll go'. So he, he says, when you've had enough cuddles. He just gets up and goes on the floor. I don't know. He thinks, well, that's it. I've done my job. And I don't understand how he knows why I'm

> sad, but he knows, he knows completely when he just needs to put his head on my lap and say, 'Mommy, I'm here', you know?
>
> But I had noticed he won't go into Henry's room now. I'll go in and polish it, but he, Uno sits outside the door, but it won't actually get in. Never settles in that room now. And he used to settle all the time when Henry was there. I think it's too sad for him.

To conclude, we asked Anne about how her relationship with Uno differed from the relationships to the two companion dogs she had before. Anne replied:

> It's just that he cares. He's just here. He's just my little boy. Maybe it's the boy that's, you know, transferred one love to another. It's just, he knows me so well and I know him so well. As I said before, he's the reason I got now because I've got no other reason you know, so. And he's just such a special dog. It's the intuitiveness of him it feels beyond his training, I think.

Conclusion

We have covered a lot of ground in this chapter. First, we have critiqued the 'standard paradigm' in dementia for its continued reliance upon human exceptionalist understandings of personhood. We then considered embodiment in dementia as an inherently multi-species phenomenon, and how a reframing of embodied personhood, away from the notion of the *Sovereign Self* towards that of the holobiont, creates new opportunities for recognising personhood and for responding to the presence of dementia. We then turned towards exploring multi-species relations between bodies. Drawing on Clifton Bryant's notion of the 'zoological dimension' we considered the ways in which interactions involving people with dementia and animals have the potential to produce more than a sense of pleasure, wellbeing or joy. What they have the potential to create is a mutual and multi-species *Being-in-the-World* within which both the person with dementia and the animal *Other* can affect and become affected by each other. This led us to an ethic of response-ability; a normative framework which recognises the potential for humans and animals to render each other capable of responding to the challenges, and opportunities, which the dementia journey typically presents. Drawing on Anne's experiences of a caring triangle, involving Anne, her late husband Henry and Uno, a bespoke-trained Dementia Dog, we explored some of the tangible ways in which inter-corporeality (a sharing of embodied experience) beyond species boundaries enabled both the human and canine members of the caring triad to affect the social accomplishment of Henry's personhood.

How, then, might a multi-species approach to personhood affect the development of dementia studies and the practice of person-centredness in dementia? One of the most significant contributions is that, by deconstructing the insuperable divide between humans (persons) and all other species of Being (non-persons), a multi-species view challenges the idea that dementia represents an existential threat to the personhood of an individual. In so doing, it enables us to regard the presence of dementia in new and *queer* ways; as for example, part of that which 'enables life itself to recompose under new relations of sustainability' (Shildrick, 2021: 95–96). Affecting such a shift in mindset, from a human-centric to a *zōē* -centric worldview, is a considerable undertaking. Less dramatic is that by adopting a multi-species view of personhood, we become able to see and to better understand the ways in which mundane relations between humans and animal *Others* can be incorporated within the lens of person-centredness. It challenges anthropocentric assumptions that only relations between humans matter in the social accomplishment of personhood. Thus, it invites us to revisit established concepts within the field, such as embodiment and inter-corporeality, and to apply these to an understanding of human–animal relations. We can but speculate, at this point, as to how such an approach may be applied beyond personhood and within other worlds of dementia, such as the laboratory, and to the relationships that develop between scientists, patients and experimental (animal) subjects. Based on the various contributions to this volume, we believe a multi-species view has the potential to reshape not only our understandings of personhood but to reconfigure the very idea of dementia itself.

Notes

1 http://www.greatapeproject.uk/

2 http://dementiadog.org

References

Abrams, D. (1996) *The Spell of the Sensuous: Perception and Language in a More-Than-Human World*, New York, NY: Vintage Books.

Arluke, A. and Sanders, C. (1996) *Regarding Animals*, Philadelphia, PA: Temple University Press.

Bana, B. and Cabreiro, F. (2019) 'The microbiome and aging', *Annual Review of Genetics*, 53(1): 239–261.

Barad, K. (2007) *Meeting the Universe Halfway: Quantum Physics and the Entanglement of Matter and Meaning*, Durham, NC: Duke University Press.

Bartlett, R. and O'Connor, D. (2007) 'From personhood to citizenship: Broadening the lens of the dementia debate', *Journal of Aging Studies*, 21(2): 107–118.

Bartlett, R. and O'Connor, D. (2010) *Broadening the Dementia Debate: Towards Social Citizenship*, Bristol: Policy Press.

Bozalek, V. and Zembylas, M. (2023) *Responsibility, Privileged Irresponsibility and Response-ability: Higher Education, Coloniality and Ecological Damage*, London: Palgrave Macmillan.

Bradford Dementia Group (1997) *Evaluating Dementia Care: The DCM Method*, Bradford: Bradford Dementia Group.

Braidotti, R. (2013) *The Posthuman*, Cambridge: Polity Press.

Bryant, C. (1979) 'The zoological connection: Animal-related human behavior', *Social Forces*, 58(2): 399–421.

Care Inspectorate (2018) *Animal Magic: The Benefits of Being Around and Caring for Animals Across Care Settings*, Dundee: Care Inspectorate.

Cohen, D. and Eisdorfer, C. (1986) *The Loss of Self: A Family Resource for the Care of Alzheimer's Disease and Related Disorders*, New York, NY: W.W. Norton & Company.

Crisp, A., Boschetti, C., Perry, M., Tunnacliffe, A. and Mickelm, G. (2015) 'Expression of multiple horizontally acquired genes is a hallmark of both vertebrate and invertebrate genomes', *Genome Biology*, 16: 50.

DeFalco, A. (2016) 'Beyond prosthetic memory: Posthumanism, embodiment, and caregiving robots', *Age, Culture, Humanities: An Interdisciplinary Journal*, 3(1): 1–31.

Descartes, R. (1993) *Discourse on Method and Meditations on First Philosophy*, Indianapolis, IN: Hackett.

Evans, S., Barrett, J., Mapes, N., Hennell, J., Atkinson, T., Bray, J., et al (2019) 'Connections with nature for people living with dementia', *Working with Older People*, 23(3): 142–151.

Gilbert, S., Sapp, J. and Tauber, A. (2012) 'A symbiotic view of life: We have never been individuals', *Quarterly Review of Biology*, 87(4): 325–341.

Gordon-Roth, J. (2020) 'Locke on personal identity', in E. Zalta (ed) *The Stanford Encyclopedia of Philosophy* [online]. Available from: https://plato.stanford.edu/archives/spr2020/entries/locke-personal-identity [Accessed 11 November 2020].

Gubrium, J. (1986) 'The social preservation of mind: The Alzheimer's disease experience', *Symbolic Interaction*, 9(1): 37–51.

Haraway, D. (2008) *When Species Meet*, Minneapolis, MN: University of Minnesota Press.

Haraway, D. (2016) *Staying with the Trouble: Making Kin the Chthulucene*. Durham NC: Duke University Press.

Hulko, W. (2004) *Dementia and Intersectionality: Exploring the Experiences of Older People with Dementia and their Significant Others*, unpublished PhD thesis, University of Stirling.

Jenkins, N., Ritchie, L. and Quinn, S. (2021) 'From reflection to diffraction: Exploring the use of vignettes within post-humanist and multi species research', *Qualitative Research*, 21(6): 975–989.

Kellert, S. (1993) 'The biological basis for human values of nature', in S. Kellert and E. Wilson (eds) *The Biophilia Hypothesis*, Washington, DC: Island Press, pp 42–69.
Kitwood, T. (1997) *Dementia Reconsidered: The Person Comes First*, Buckingham: Open University Press.
Kitwood, T. and Bredin, K. (1992) 'Towards a theory of dementia care: Personhood and well-being', *Ageing & Society*, 12(3): 269–287.
Kontos, P. (2005) 'Embodied selfhood in Alzheimer's disease: Rethinking person centred care', *Dementia*, 4(4): 553–570.
Levinson, B. (1972) *Pets and Human Development*, Springfield, IL: Charles C. Thomas.
Malcolm, R., Ecks, S. and Pickersgill, M. (2018) '"It just opens up their world": Autism, empathy, and the therapeutic effects of equine interactions', *Anthropology & Medicine*, 25(2): 220–234.
Merleau-Ponty, M. (1968) *The Visible and the Invisible: Followed by Working Notes*, Evanston, IL: Northwestern University Press.
Nhat Hanh, T. (1991) *Peace is Every Step: The Path of Mindfulness in Everyday Life*, Ashland, OR: Blackstone Publishing.
Nhat Hanh, T. (2017) *The Art of Living: Peace and Freedom in the Here and Now*, New York, NY: HarperCollins.
Nolan, M., Davies, S., Brown, J., Keady, J. and Nolan, J. (2004) 'Beyond person-centred care: A new vision for gerontological nursing', *Journal of Clinical Nursing*, 13(1): 45–53.
Pinel, P. (1806) *A Treatise on Insanity*, London: Messrs, Cadell and Davies.
Quinn, J. and Blandon, C. (2017) 'The potential for lifelong learning in dementia: A post-humanist exploration', *International Journal of Lifelong Education*, 36(5): 578–594.
Quinn, J. and Blandon, C. (2020) *Lifelong Learning and Dementia: A Posthumanist Perspective*, London: Palgrave Macmillan.
Reiger, S. and Bolinski, I. (2020) 'Beyond the anthropocene: Are we entering a "multispecies turn"?', *Scientia*. doi: 10.33548/SCIENTIA499
Ritchie, L., Quinn, S., Tolson, D., Jenkins, N. and Sharp, B. (2021) 'Exposing the mechanisms underlying successful animal-assisted interventions for people with dementia: A realistic evaluation of the Dementia Dog project', *Dementia*, 20(1): 66–83.
Sabat, S. and Harré, R. (1992) 'The construction and deconstruction of self in Alzheimer's disease', *Ageing and Society*, 12(4): 443–461.
Sagan, D. and Margulis, L. (1993) 'God, Gaia, and biophilia', in S. Kellert and E. Wilson (eds) *The Biophilia Hypothesis*, Washington, DC: Island Press, pp 345–364.
Sagan, L. (1967) 'On the origin of mitosing cells', *Journal of Theoretical Biology*, 14(3): 225–274.

Shildrick, M. (2021) 'Queering dementia: Technologies, visceral prostheses and embodiment', *Lambda Nordica*, 26(2–3): 76–101.

Sweeting, H. and Gilhooly, M. (1997) 'Dementia and the phenomenon of social death', *Sociology of Health & Illness*, 12(3): 93–117.

Tronto, J. (1993) *Moral Boundaries: A Political Argument for an Ethic of Care*, New York, NY: Routledge.

Twigg, J. (2010) 'Clothing and dementia: A neglected dimension?', *Journal of Aging Studies*, 24(4): 223–230.

Twigg, J., Wolkowitz, C., Cohen, R. and Nettleton, S. (2011) 'Conceptualising body work in health and social care', *Sociology of Health & Illness*, 33(2): 171–188.

Ulrich, R. (1993) 'Biophilia, biophobia, and natural landscapes', in S. Kellert and E. Wilson (eds) *The Biophilia Hypothesis*, Washington, DC: Island Press, pp 73–137.

Wilson, E. (1993) 'Biophilia and the conservation ethic', in S. Kellert and E. Wilson (eds) *The Biophilia Hypothesis*, Washington, DC: Island Press, pp 31–41.

Wilson, R. (1984) *Biophilia: The Human Bond with Other Species*, Cambridge, MA: Harvard University Press.

Wolfe, C. (2003) *Animal Rites: American Culture, the Discourse of Species, and Posthumanist Theory*, Chicago, IL: University of Chicago Press.

Wolfe, C. (2010) *What is Posthumanism?*, Minneapolis, MN: University of Minnesota Press.

Yakimicki, M., Edwards, N., Richards, E. and Beck, A. (2019) 'Animal-assisted intervention and dementia: A systematic review', *Clinical Nursing Research*, 28(1): 9–29.

8

Forging human–animal bonds? Introducing robotic pets into the care of people with dementia

Ann M. Toohey, Jayne Beselt, Jennifer Hewson, David B. Hogan and Melanie Rock

Introduction

They have arrived. Since first appearing on the market in 2015, Joy for All™ animatronic dogs and cats (Figure 8.1), and more recently birds, have been promoted as intriguing, affordable, effective devices that can improve quality of life for older adults, particularly those experiencing cognitive deficits and dementias (Aging and Health Technology Watch, 2020). They can be conveniently acquired via the Internet and at a reasonable cost for many (that is, <US$150).[1] Moreover, the campaign for these 'robotic' pets, and for those of other manufacturers, has been an unquestionable success. Sales of Joy for All™ robotic pets have surpassed a half-million units (Ageless Innovation, 2022) while worldwide, robotic dog sales alone increased by over 16 per cent in 2022 (Technavio, 2022). As the figures attest, these interactive devices can be found in both private homes and care facilities with increasing frequency. Even mass media has been captivated by this trend, as exemplified by an extensive *New Yorker* magazine article that explored the robotic pets phenomenon in 'What robots can – and can't – do for the old and lonely' (Engelhart, 2021).

The idea of robotic animal interventions to enhance quality of life for people living with dementia is not new, nor was it when the Joy for All™ pets were first introduced. The PARO baby harp seal robot was launched in 2003 as an alternative to animal-assisted therapies for people living with dementia in settings where live animals were not practical (Shibata et al, 2005).[2] The hope was that PARO would have a therapeutic impact similar to the promising outcomes of live animal-assisted interactions for people living with dementia (Jenkins et al, 2021). PARO has now gone through eight design generations and there have been multiple studies exploring its effectiveness for a range of outcomes, including agitation, depression, emotional benefits and overall engagement (Moyle et al, 2017; Minmin

Figure 8.1: 2022 models of Joy for All™ robotic puppy and kitten

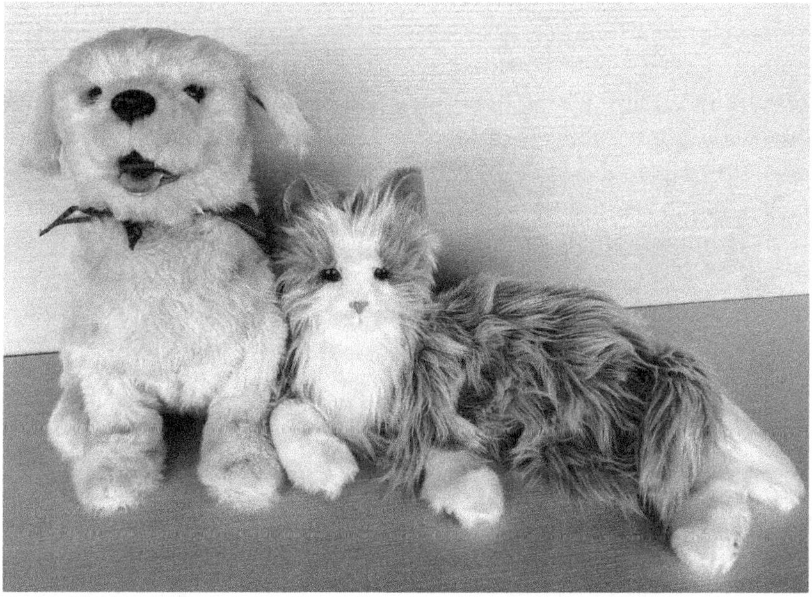

Source: Photo by A.M. Toohey

et al, 2019). Some researchers have also sought to understand the ethics of introducing PARO into care settings for people living with dementia, and have noted the ethical complexities of promoting human–robotic animal interactions for this population (Sharkey and Wood, 2014; Chiberska, 2018).

Despite its technological advancements, research evidence and therapeutic potential, PARO – with a price tag of ~US$6,000 – has not become a standard therapeutic tool used in most care facilities. However, use of Joy for All™ robotic pets appears to be on the rise (Aging and Health Technology Watch, 2020). Researchers' attention has naturally followed this movement towards integrating the more affordable robotic dog and cat models into care delivery, particularly for people living with different stages of dementia (Koh et al, 2021). Studies to date have focused on the therapeutic impact of robotic pet interventions on a number of treatment outcomes, as well as on implementation considerations (Koh et al, 2022; Nelson and Westenskow, 2022). Even as this literature continues to grow, however, less scholarly attention has been paid to social and relational dimensions of human–robotic pet interactions and the opportunities for personhood and self-expression that they may facilitate.

Our research team became curious about the nature of interactions with the Joy for All™ robotic pets by older adults living with dementia and the perspectives of formal (professional) and family caregivers. In this chapter we present observations regarding this phenomenon. While other objects of attachment could arguably be considered, the Joy for All™ robotic animals piqued our interest due to their reliance on new, albeit simple, technologies (for example, touch sensors that activate a response), growing popularity, theoretical links to multi-species and posthumanism scholarship, and the current lag in understanding how the therapeutic and social implications of this growing phenomenon are intertwined. As a sidenote, in this chapter we do not compare live and robotic animal interventions. We note that this is an area requiring additional work, as the available literature contrasting the two is limited and somewhat inconclusive (examples include Kramer et al, 2009; Marx et al, 2010; Valentí Soler et al, 2015; Thodberg et al, 2016a; 2016b). It does appear, though, that robotic pets and live animals may both have similar abilities to stimulate interactions with persons living with dementia (Moyle et al, 2017).

Theoretical considerations

Our study was guided by a belief that therapeutic interest in and work with robotic pets may have relevance within a relationship-centred care framework (Nolan et al, 2004). Relationship-centred care recognises the multiple overlapping relationships that shape care provision, and that include care-related interactions among people living with dementia, professional staff, family and a wider community (Nolan et al, 2004). While we assume that care delivery is primarily directed at the person living with dementia, robotic pets may also create opportunities for those living with dementia to experience caring activities aimed at these interactive entities. Promoting opportunities to express these types of caring behaviours may also support dignity of identity, that is, one's relational status as reflecting one's past and possible future, as reinforced by interactions with others (Cruise and Lashewicz, 2022), for people living with dementia.

We also believe that human–robotic pet relationships merit exploration using a posthumanism lens. In proposing a critical posthumanist approach to dementia care, Jenkins (2017) observes that our humanist episteme may be responsible for many assumptions around the deficiencies of people living with dementia. This focus on deficiencies, we suggest, may lead to those living with dementia being excluded from opportunities to provide care. Jenkins further suggests that 'critical posthumanism seeks to develop new ways of thinking about persons and personhood in ways that address humanism's in-built tendencies to order sentient beings hierarchically' (Jenkins, 2017: 1494). Hierarchical ordering may be also reflected in conventional views on what constitute meaningful interactions for humans to engage in and with whom or what (Shildrick, 2021). These views may underlie some of the critiques on the ethics of using robotic pets for people living with dementia (Sparrow, 2002; Sharkey and Wood, 2014; Chiberska, 2018), yet the popularity of their use among people living with dementia continues to grow. Drawing upon posthumanism when considering these tensions may help us to garner new insights into this somewhat divisive phenomenon.

DeFalco (2020: 33) also highlights the complexities around acceptance of relationships of care between human beings and robots, given the perpetuation of 'a wilfully anthropocentric perspective that makes "real" or "authentic" care the exclusive domain of human animals'. DeFalco focuses on care relationships between humans and human-like robots or androids, yet we extend this work by considering non-human robotic animals as prospective recipients of care and affection offered by people living with dementia. Caring for others – including non-human companion animals – is both a valued occupation and a means of promoting health and wellbeing for *both* the care provider and recipient (Zimolag and Krupa, 2009; Rock, 2017; Toohey et al, 2017; Toohey, 2023). Furthermore, the relational opportunities proffered by robotic pets may also enable 'contact with their previous sense of self' (Shildrick, 2021: 78), which, as discussed earlier, can promote dignity of identity (Cruise and Lashewicz, 2022) via a sense of continuity, specifically for those people living with dementia who demonstrate an affinity for the robotic pets.

Methodology

We adopted an ethnographic approach (Stewart, 1998) to gain a rich, *in situ* understanding of ways that robotic pets may be influencing care practices and social dynamics within settings where care is being provided to people living with dementia. We were unable to conduct extensive observational fieldwork due to restricted access in response to the onset of the COVID-19 pandemic. Instead, we relied primarily on data collected via semi-structured interviews that sampled a range of both formal care providers (for example, paid staff or clinicians working within continuing care; staff within community organisations) and family caregivers for people living with dementia. As vaccinations were introduced and restrictions were reduced, members of our research team conducted observational work within a facility-based care setting. These observations helped to triangulate and enrich our understanding of the interview data, informing our analysis. Ethics certification for our study was received from our local institutional ethics review board (REB 20–2089).

Participants and research setting

We recruited participants (n=17) purposively to attain multiple perspectives on experiences with introducing robotic pets to people living with dementia. Prospective study participants were identified through our research team's professional (n=14) and personal networks (n=1), media coverage (n=1) and referral from other study participants (n=1). Most participants were women (n=15). Overall, we recruited participants involved primarily in formal care provision within congregate care settings (n=13), community programmes that used or were considering introducing robotic pets (n=2) and family caregivers (n=2). Two participants held multiple perspectives, being both family caregivers of people living with dementia and having professional roles that involved robotic pets. Many of the formal care providers also reflected upon direct experiences of families whose loved ones were living with dementia, but who were not participants in this study. These views nonetheless helped to inform our understanding of a wide range of experiences with robotic pets.

Most of our participants lived and worked in our local setting (that is, Calgary, n=10) or within our Canadian province (that is, Alberta, n=5). One participant was located elsewhere in Canada, while another was involved in facility-based care delivery in the United States. Because of the widespread popularity of Joy for All™ robotic pets in North America and elsewhere, we did not use geographical location as a reason to exclude participation in our study. An overview of participants is presented in Table 8.1.

Interviews and observational work

Semi-structured ethnographic interviews (Spradley, 1979) and observational field work (Emerson et al, 1995) took place between March 2021 and August 2022. Interviews were designed to elucidate participants' care provider roles and explore direct experiences with people living with dementia and robotic pets.

The interviews considered in this analysis were either individual (n=9) or group interviews with between two and six participants (n=3). Four of the participants were involved in two progressive group interviews, each scheduled a month apart, to garner insights prior to and following the introduction of Joy for All™ robotic pets into their recreation programming. In addition to this study, this latter series of group interviews is informing the development of recommendations for staff working with robotic pets within formal care settings.

All interviews but one were conducted by the lead author (AT), typically with another team member present (JB or else research assistants AB or BF – see Acknowledgements). The other interview was conducted by another author (MR) supported by research assistant AB (see Acknowledgements). Most interviews were conducted using videoconferencing software (that is, Zoom) or telephone, though two group interviews with members of a recreation therapy team were conducted in person once pandemic-related visiting and gathering restrictions had eased.

Between the two in-person interviews, a research assistant (BF – see Acknowledgements) had the opportunity to observe two different recreation

Table 8.1: Description of study participants

Pseudonym	Role(s)	Gender	Location
P1	Community organisation Family care provider (son)	M	Eastern Canada
P2	Formal care provider (physician)	M	Calgary
P3	Formal care provider (nurse)	F	Calgary
P4	Community organisation	F	Alberta
P5	Family care provider (daughter)	F	Alberta
P6	Formal care provider (comfort care aide)	F	Calgary
P7	Formal care provider (nurse)	F	USA
P8	Formal care provider (recreation therapist)	F	Alberta
P9	Family care provider (daughter) Community organisation	F	Calgary
P10	Formal care provider (nurse)	F	Alberta
P11	Formal care provider (recreation therapist)	F	Alberta
P12*	Formal care provider (recreation therapist)	F	Calgary
P13*	Formal care provider (recreation therapist)	F	Calgary
P14*	Formal care provider (recreation therapy assistant)	F	Calgary
P15*	Formal care provider (recreation therapy assistant)	F	Calgary
P16	Formal care provider (recreation therapy assistant)	F	Calgary
P17	Formal care provider (recreation therapy assistant)	F	Calgary

Note: * Interviewed as a group at two different times, approximately one month apart.

therapists introducing robotic pets to long-term care residents living with dementia. Extensive field notes were taken, and observed interactions were discussed both with the lead author (AT) and then during the second group interview with this team, which helped address both respondent validation and researcher objectivity (Stewart, 1998).

Following each interview, the researcher(s) involved prepared reflexive written research memos to capture initial impressions, also considering both similarities and differences within the growing corpus of collected interview data. All interviews with one exception were recorded and transcribed. For this exception, which was an individual interview, extensive notes were taken and the record of the interview was approved by the participant.

Analysis

Our initial analysis was inductive but guided by our interest in social dynamics linked to the use of robotic pets in care settings. The lead author

(AT) and second author (JB) led the thematic analysis, initially identifying broad themes. As our understanding evolved, we made comparisons across interviews to understand both converging and diverging perspectives and experiences. Early insights were discussed with the rest of the research team as we sought to consider the genesis of the different perspectives shared by study participants, in relation to their roles in care delivery. As a final analytic step, we considered the theoretical frames, including posthumanism care (Jenkins, 2017; DeFalco, 2020) and relational care (Nolan et al, 2004). Further discussion took place with all authors prior to finalising our analysis.

Findings

While the 17 participants brought multiple vantages to our study, we were struck by three key themes within our interview data that offered insights into the nature of interactions catalysed by robotic pets. The first, *reluctant acquiescence*, dealt with the challenges in accepting the possibility that the eventual reality of a person living with dementia might include attachment to a robotic pet. The second, *meaningful utility*, underscored ways that many participants embraced the practical usefulness of Joy for All™ robotic pets as a therapeutic modality that could enhance quality of life for residents living with dementia by introducing meaningful personal experiences into their daily lives. The final theme, *navigating illusion and risk*, described both the benefits and risks associated with enabling robotic pet relationships for people living with dementia and the lengths sometimes taken to facilitate these relationships.

Reluctant acquiescence

Reluctant acquiescence was most often expressed by family caregivers. This theme generally captures the temporal progression of reactions to robotic pets in the context of both coming to terms with a parent's or spouse's diagnosis and adapting to the disease's progression. It also touches on discomfort with how a person living with dementia might be perceived if they form a close bond with a robotic animal. A compelling discussion of this progression was shared during our interview with P5. P5's mother had gradually lost the ability to care for a (living) pet dog who she and her husband had been allowed to keep when they moved into a congregate care setting. Her cognitive state rapidly declined, and P5 began noticing things that concerned her related to the dog's health and wellbeing. With her father's agreement, P5 decided not to return the dog to her parents' apartment within the facility following an outdoor walk and took it home with her instead. 'It was absolutely necessary.' While her mother noticed the dog's absence the following day, her questioning about the dog's whereabouts did not persist or seem distressful.

As her mother's condition declined further, a member of the care team suggested that P5 consider purchasing her mother a Joy for All™ robotic dog, which P5 thought sounded 'quite frankly a little ridiculous for someone who had a real pet for so many years'. Still, she acquiesced. With considerable emotion, P5 described her deep disappointment when facility staff presented her mother with the robotic dog, which had arrived in the post, without P5 being present. 'Do [they] have any idea how rare those occasions of joy are that [they] just robbed me of?'

When asked how this new relationship was being received by care staff, she said 'Well, it's kind of them to recognise that she is deriving some element of pleasure from having this robot, and so that would seem to be good news, because there doesn't seem to be a great deal that makes her smile or elicit a more normal response from her.' P5 was sceptical, though, that her mother would miss the robotic dog if it were to disappear, and wondered 'Out of sight, out of mind?' Even so, she was resolved that the robotic dog would remain with her mother even as she transitioned into a room within the memory care wing of the facility.

The underlying scepticism regarding the meaning of a robotic pet to a person living with dementia recurred in other interviews. P9, for instance, reflected upon her family's experiences, having introduced a robotic cat into her mother's life shortly after the initial diagnosis of dementia several years prior. P9, who was also involved with dementia advocacy, had been aware of the new Joy for All™ product and suggested to other family members that one be purchased for her mother. Her mother had grown up with a cat, and P9 wondered whether introducing the robotic cat early enough during her illness might lead her mother to form an attachment to it. Her father resisted, in P9's words, because it was 'infantilising' and because 'he didn't want to think that she was going to get to the point where this would be a normal thing, right?' However, as her mother's dementia progressed and care needs intensified, P9 described how her father began to see the value in it, as an object that attracted her mother through its movements and sounds. The robotic cat held her attention and petting the cat calmed her when she was upset. P9 also shared her view that:

> [A]nything that provides any kind of comfort and calm is great, as far as I'm concerned. My brother less so. [Interviewer: He doesn't like watching her with the cat? It bothers him?] A little bit. I would say he definitely thinks that they should have a [live or real] dog that she could actually interact with, which they cannot because [it would be] one more thing on my dad's plate.

P9 also queried the extent to which removing the robotic cat from her mother's life would have any impact: 'So it's not an "Oh where's the cat today?" If it's gone it's gone, there's no memory of it at all.'

On the other hand, P8, a formal care provider, described during our interview a situation where the wife of a resident living with dementia struggled to accept her husband's attachment to a robotic dog, which had been employed to mitigate responsive behaviours he was experiencing:

> [H]is wife didn't understand why someone would want a robotic pet. Or didn't understand why it would bring so much joy, especially when she has a [live] dog. And when she'd bring the dog [to visit], he was so fascinated with the robotic dog that he just wasn't interested in the real dog. But, yeah, she had taken [away] the one [robotic] pet, so we ended up losing [it] because we didn't have the buy-in for it. We managed to get him another [robotic] pet later, which was amazing because he was so happy again … and I think she's been able to see the joy that it brought him, so I think she kind of came around.

Reluctance to accept the idea of a robotic pet was not wholly limited to family members. One formal care provider, P7, was firmly opposed to the therapeutic use of robotic pets:

> I won't dispute the studies that demonstrate that when someone has been agitated and you give them that robotic cat, they're going to respond. But I just come back to that place where, what have we done? How did we see that person? How do caregivers see that person? Do they see them as 'less than'? And in that devaluation and that 'less than dignified' approach to what we're doing, have we somehow put something in that care partner's mind, where we are fuelling the devaluation that comes with the diagnosis of dementia? And again, it really is how we see that person … as a society if we are trying to destigmatise those that are living with dementia, if we are trying to create dementia inclusivity, I think this is contrary.

For P7, the therapeutic potential of robotic pets is of less consequence than the potential harm caused by her perception of the indignity with which others may view human–robotic animal interactions.

Meaningful utility

While acknowledging that robotic pets do not appeal to *all* residents (or families), the existential struggle towards acceptance of a bond between a person and a robotic pet was largely absent from those delivering care professionally, as well as for those considering robotic pets during the later stage of dementia progression. Interest in and support for Joy for All™ pets was predominant, and they were described as offering both therapeutic utility and other positive experiences for many residents. There was often a sense that encounters with robotic pets led to meaningful engagement for these residents:

> In those who appreciated the cats, it was a calming presence for them, and they could pet it. And the fact that it moved a little bit, and it was something to hold, and it kept them from fidgeting and rummaging. So, there's that kind of physical component to it, but there's also the psychological component of having companionship, right? (P2)

For some, companionship led to engaging in acts of pet care, as would be done for a live companion animal:

> I had all the [Joy for All™] cats up top and you can see them, and she's very well aware that they aren't real. I gave her one and she's had it now for three weeks and she talks to it, pets it. She takes very, very good care of it. Gives it water … brush[es] it. She is just very thankful to have a companion when there's nobody in her room. (P13)

For some, however, the demands of pet care caused some stress. P9 reflected of her mother: '[S]ometimes she's worried about it, where its water is, and where its food is … and sometimes we'll be having dinner and she'll say "Oh, we need to feed the cat".'

Opportunities to provide this type of care were also effective for engaging long-term care residents who otherwise might not have taken an interest in the robotic pets. P14 shared: '[M]y go-to approach that I find is successful is, usually I'd say, "Oh, hey, can you please do me a favour? I need to go and do something. Would you mind watching my cat for me?" And I've never gotten a no.' P14 also recognised how creating a meaningful and constructive role for residents living with dementia also offered an opportunity for them to feel useful and capable: '[With the robotic cat] they're like: "She's lying on me. She likes what I'm doing. She's going backwards, lifting the paw. I'm doing something right." Yeah.'

Many participants identified understanding past experiences of residents as a strategy for determining who might benefit from spending time with a robotic pet. Some care providers noted, however, that a history of pets was not necessarily a prerequisite to engaging with robotic pets:

> I think at the start we had said that [life history] would be super important. We have to know their life history. But now … just because

> their life history or assessment doesn't tell you that they had cats all their life doesn't mean that they're not going to respond well to this cat. So, my opinion on that one has shifted. (P12)

Most formal care providers in our sample felt that bringing robotic pets into their facilities had enhanced their ability to promote quality of life. And while other objects like dolls and stuffed animals have long been common fixtures within care facilities that support people living with dementia, there was a sense that Joy for All™ robotic pets offered something more. One participant explained, 'I think they're more universally accepted' (P10). Another shared: 'Some residents might have had a teddy bear or something, they just like that for their security or comfort. But this has really been the first time that I've got to see such positive benefit from specifically those animated dogs' (P8).

Many formal care providers also mentioned family members' interests in robotic pets after they witnessed their use in facilities. For instance, P12 reflected that 'We even had a family email us that they saw one of the [care team members] doing this with the robotic pet and ask, "Can you get them to try it with my husband? And then if he responds, let me know and I'll buy him one".' It seemed that family caregivers were able to accept the meaningful utility of robotic pets if they were introduced at an advanced dementia stage rather than at an earlier one. For instance, P1 described his mother's transition into a residential care setting:

> When she had to go into the [nursing] home during COVID, I did purchase her one. … What I can't get over is as soon as [the Joy for All™ cat] meows, it doesn't matter. She can be complaining to me, and saying, 'I want to die.' And then that cat will meow, and she'll turn around and just start laughing and then the whole mood changes.

Similarly, as caregiving demands evolved in response to disease progression, a robotic pet could offer respite. As P9 shared, reflecting on her father's caregiver role for her mother: '[The robotic cat is] something that will take her attention a little bit and that's nice for him, because he sometimes would just like to watch the News, right?'

Navigating illusion and risk

While most of the family caregivers we spoke with expressed ambivalence or discomfort with reinforcing a loved one's attachment to a robotic pet, most of the formal care providers we spoke with had little compunction with perpetuating the illusion that the robotic pet was a real animal, when the situation called for it. They felt this strategy helped sustain the therapeutic utility of the devices and could also help mitigate risks of harm to a resident. For example, P12 described a resident who was so attached to his robotic dog that he tried to carry it under his arm wherever he went, while also using a mobility aid. To mitigate his risk of falling, P12 reflected:

> [You need to] be aware of your surroundings and just think fast. … I know an animal has to go outside and go to the bathroom. That's how I'm going to try and redirect this resident. … 'Oh, they need to go to the bathroom right now. Let's put them down on the grass while we walk.' They think it's real. So, you think it's real.

Managing this illusion was less straightforward in situations where a person living with dementia was experiencing shifting perceptions about the robotic pet:

> I did see one resident that within a ten-minute interaction with the [robotic] cat, they were cognitively flip-flopping minute by minute between 'the cat is real, the cat's a fake'. And that was perplexing to watch and hear her verbalise 'Well, it's just a robot, it's just a toy', and then start talking about what it's doing, as a real cat. (P10)

Participants often found themselves balancing efforts to sustain the illusion of reality for one resident while acknowledging the cognitive capacity of other residents who recognised the animal as being robotic. These discontinuities in perceptions were recognised as potential sources of conflict and confusion among residents. P6, for instance, discussed strategies for defraying such tensions between residents through direct conversation and acknowledgement: 'I know it's not real, you know it's not real, but it helps them.' A subtle non-verbal exchange was also sometimes used to balance the interests of both residents in such cases:

> If [you're] more cognitively intact, you don't want somebody coming to you with some robotic cat pretending it's real. That could be a bit offensive. And so, you know, a quick wink in their direction would be that acknowledgment that 'Don't worry. We're not going to do this to you'. (P10)

Sometimes, however, mitigation of differing perceptions was more complicated, as care providers sought to balance the risks and benefits of attachment to a robotic pet:

> So, this gentleman wanted to hold his [robotic] dog and stand up at the same time. So, I had to get his permission. 'Can I please hold your dog

> while you stand up?' I held his dog and his neighbour got very angry that I was holding the dog and hit me. And she was saying 'That's his dog' and I shouldn't have that dog. … We had to navigate that, but [it was] something I also wasn't expecting. (P12)

In some situations, the risks associated with strong attachments were determined to be too substantial to navigate through reinforcing the illusion. P9 recounted one such situation: '[H]e would be aggressive about [his robotic dog], physically aggressive … he ended up in the hospital for a short amount of time and [hospital staff] said 'No, we're not dealing with this.' And then the family chose not to reintroduce it because it was too difficult.' In this case, the utility of the robotic pet was outweighed by the risks of harm and conflict linked to the robotic pet. And yet, P10 was somewhat more circumspect about this type of situation: 'We have some residents that go through a phase of paranoia and possessiveness. … I would say if not the [robotic] cat, it would be a different item.'

Discussion

This study sought to explore the social and relational care dimensions of the use of Joy for All™ pets with older adults living with dementia. In doing this, we were interested in learning more about how use of robotic pets may influence caregiving in ways that extend beyond their therapeutic utility. We were also inspired to better understand the ethical tensions around the use of robotic pets, which raise questions around their appropriateness even as their therapeutic potential holds promise. In what follows, we consider both critical posthumanism scholarship and a relationship-centred care framework for their theoretical insights into this increasingly popular phenomenon.

The findings presented within the *reluctant acquiescence* theme highlight the possibility of discomfort with the notion that a person could form a strong attachment to a robotic pet, which was felt by some to be both undignified and infantilising. Linked to the sense of discomfort, we also detected ambivalence about introducing the robotic pet in the first place, even as the benefits become apparent. To interpret this discomfort, we return to DeFalco's discussion of the roles of social robots from a posthumanist care perspective. Witnessing an older person experiencing an emotional connection with an inorganic entity like a Joy for All™ robotic pet may create an internalised struggle to cross what DeFalco (2020: 48) defines as 'false boundaries between a multitude of human/non-human ontologies'. We would further distinguish, however, organic versus inorganic non-human ontologies as being at the root of our troubling. When we exclude people living with dementia from opportunities to care for things, such as an organic (living) non-human animal (that is, a pet) out of concern for its welfare, we may fail to recognise how the loss of a caregiving role can also exclude the person from opportunities for self-expression and engagement in meaningful roles.

From within a humanist ontology, the futility of providing care to something that doesn't require it, such as a robotic pet, may account for the resistance to accepting robotic pets that was shared by several participants, primarily family members. We also wonder if this resistance represents a distinction between families viewing robotic pets as replacements for live companion animals rather than as therapeutic tools that contribute to quality of life. When viewed through a posthumanist lens, we might focus instead on ways that these human–robot interactions can reintroduce opportunities to promote, for example, dignity of identity via spontaneous acts of caring for and experiencing companionship with a robotic animal (Sharkey and Wood, 2014; Chiberska, 2018). While acknowledging the illusion of agency conveyed by robotic pets, Shildrick (2021: 81) also observes that 'they do generate very real responses and effects, both emotional and somatic, and that alone unsettles and queers the confines of the human'. Robotic pets may represent an avenue through which those living with dementia might be afforded opportunities to participate in posthumanist care, as being 'vital, vibrant relationality produced by and through the constant flux of tools and technologies' (DeFalco, 2020: 51).

The 'vibrant relationality' highlighted by DeFalco is also well aligned with perspectives represented within the *meaningful utility* theme. The safe creation of opportunities for people with reduced cognitive faculties to engage in caring and affectionate behaviours with robotic pets were generally recognised as beneficial by nearly all the formal care providers participating in this study. Thus, opportunities for creating bonds between residents and robotic pets were often forged with intention. Connections between people living with dementia and robotic pets served the relational interests of the person involved, the care staff and family members, by offering respite from states of agitation, depression, boredom and loneliness while also giving way to companionship, caregiving and purpose. The interactive response to attention by the robotic pets, through sensor-activated vocalisations and movements, may elicit a sense of agency and reconnection with former sense of self that is rarely experienced as dementia progresses. If we are able to refrain from defining hierarchical categorisations around who or what constitute appropriate dyads in caring relationships, then the focus can shift onto the value of a meaningful interaction for the person living with dementia (Shildrick, 2021), rather than quibbling about the illusion that sparks an empathetic response.

This critical posthumanism interpretation of the meaningful utility of robotic pets can also be linked with relationship-centred care, particularly as described by Nolan et al (2004: 50) in a 'Senses Framework'. According to the Senses Framework, relational care creates for the care recipient senses of security, continuity, belonging, purpose, achievement and significance (Nolan et al, 2004). As apparent in our data, each of these 'senses' was supported through engaged interactions with robotic pets. For instance, security and continuity were potentially generated through recognising and leveraging individuals' personal histories and former relationships with pets, though we also acknowledge that the utility of robotic pets did not necessarily hinge on past pet relationships. Senses of belonging, purpose, achievement and significance were also manifest when interactions were presented as opportunities to assist staff as well as to 'take care of' the robotic pet in ways that were both valuable and meaningful. Engaging residents with robotic pets can elevate the social relationship between the professional caregiver, a person living with dementia, and a robotic pet beyond being simply participation or interaction facilitated only with the intention of keeping a resident engaged or distracted.

Critical posthumanism may also be helpful for considering *navigating illusion and risk*. Just as Jenkins (2017: 1491) troubles the perpetuation of 'hierarchical orderings based on binary distinctions' including 'natural-artificial, human-non-human', we grapple with the tension between actively encouraging activities that some view as demeaning and undignified and, on the other hand, enabling the many positive outcomes that were described throughout our interviews and in the literature (Koh et al, 2021). Negative responses to the prospective illusion of sentience that may be perpetuated by Joy for All™ robotic pets may reflect the humanist distinctions between 'natural-artificial, human-non-human' at play during human–robotic pet interactions. From the critical posthumanist perspective, though, recognising opportunities for meaningful self-expression and dignity of identity created by the interactive Joy for All™ robotic pets might serve as counterpoints to such contentions of deceptiveness and infantilisation of using these devices. By softening the binary distinctions around the acceptability of relational experiences with 'artificial' animals, we might also create space for reinforcing the illusion that a robotic pet merits care as a means of mitigating the risks that emerge from stronger attachments that some people living with dementia have to their robotic pets. Even as our study alerts us to situations where the potential harms of the human–robotic animal interaction may outweigh the benefits, we wonder whether creative approaches to leveraging rather than disrupting the illusion might effectively be used to diffuse outbursts reflecting paranoia and distrust. This supposition has also been considered by Shildrick (2021: 83), who describes the unwelcome and anger-inducing 'withdrawal' of robotic animals from engaged residents as an 'ethical misstep'.

Our findings confirm that involving robotic pets in care delivery for people living with dementia can be a relational phenomenon with broad social implications, rather than simply a therapeutic tool. Our participants described how robotic pets may serve purposes that extend beyond the dyad of the person living with dementia and a robotic pet. Might robotic pets, then, be an 'instrument of control' (Jenkins et al, 2021), employed to assuage responsive behaviours through the guise of offering comfort and agency to people living with dementia living in facilities? While none of the formal care providers we spoke to discussed ways that robotic pets made their own work easier, responsive behaviours were nonetheless mentioned at times as an impetus for introducing a robotic pet to a specific resident. Yet several participants also described their willingness to creatively adapt strategies to preserve positive experiences for *all* residents, including those who did not wish to interact with them. Even for family caregivers, the invaluable respite that a robotic pet sometimes offered was framed as a secondary rather than primary benefit of enabling the bond between a person living with dementia and a robotic pet.

We acknowledge some ontological and methodological limitations to our study, particularly in not involving people living with dementia as research participants. We were not able to garner their experiences with the relational and social dimensions of interacting with robotic pets. Instead, we relied on the perspectives of those who decide when, if and with whom a robotic pet might be shared. This power imbalance asserts a level of control within the social setting and may also compromise personal agency and self-determination of the relationship for people living with dementia. While we had opportunities to observe people living with dementia interacting with Joy for All™ cats, our understandings of these interactions were interpretative, as our focus was on the social component of delivery in eliciting a positive, neutral or negative response. Future studies might aspire to gain a better understanding of ways the recipients of the intervention experience robotic pets by appropriately involving people living with dementia (Webb et al, 2020).

Conclusion

We tentatively conclude that the growing popularity of introducing Joy for All™ robotic pets to people living with dementia may be understood as a merging of the 'multi-species approach to care and caring' (Jenkins et al, 2021: 3) with an advancement of the concept of critical posthumanist care for people living with dementia (Jenkins, 2017; DeFalco, 2020). We recommend that these theories, alongside an evolving conception of relational care that engages with dignity of identity, might guide future explorations into the social, practical and therapeutic study of this contemporary phenomenon.

Throughout our analysis, we have been inspired by Jenkins' (2017: 1493) posthumanism challenge, 'to question and problematise the underlying assumptions upon which contemporary models of care are based'. Should a humanist view of robotic pets as demeaning prevail, particularly outside of the formal care sector, use of robotic pets could further stigmatise people living with dementia who form strong attachments to them. In viewing robotic pets as having an acceptable role within a critical posthumanist understanding of relationship-centred care, however, we wonder if perhaps the ontological division between dignity and indignity in caring with, caring for and caring about a robotic companion animal may be a false one.

Disclaimer

The authors were not compensated by Joy for All™ or other manufacturers of robotic pets for this work. The views expressed here solely represent the opinions of the authors.

Acknowledgements

The authors wish to acknowledge research assistants, Amberlee Boulton and Brooklynn Fernandes and Dr Cindy Adams, for their valuable contributions to this study. In-kind support was provided by the University of Calgary Brenda Strafford Centre on Aging and the Brenda Strafford Foundation. Funding support was received from the University of Calgary Brenda Strafford Foundation Chair in Geriatric Medicine held by Dr Jayna Holroyd-Leduc; a Social Sciences and Humanities Research Council of Canada (SSHRC) Partnership Engage Grant held by Dr Ann M. Toohey (File 892–2022–0013); and a Wellcome Trust Small Grants in Humanities and Social Sciences held by Dr Nicholas Jenkins (Grant Reference: WT: 218928/Z/19/Z).

Notes

1 See joyforall.com

2 www.parorobots.com

References

Ageless Innovation (2022) 'Ageless innovation celebrates half million Joy for All™ companion pets adopted by older adults', *Cision PR Web*, 1 November. Available from: https://www.prweb.com/releases/ageless-innovation-celebrates-half-million-joy-for-all-tm-companion-pets-adopted-by-older-adults-801085163.html [Accessed 1 November 2022].

Aging and Health Technology Watch (2020) *Impact and Benefit: Research Findings for Joy for All Companion Pets from Ageless Innovation.* Available from: https://www.ageinplacetech.com/files/aip/Joy%20for%20All_Impact%20and%20Benefit_Final%20May%202020.pdf [Accessed 1 November 2022].

Chiberska, D. (2018) 'The use of robotic animals in dementia care: Challenges and ethical dilemmas', *Mental Health Practice*, 21(10): 23–28.

Cruise, C.E. and Lashewicz, B.M. (2022) 'Dementia and dignity of identity: A qualitative evidence synthesis', *Dementia*, 21(4): 1233–1249.

DeFalco, A. (2020) 'Towards a theory of posthuman care: Real humans and caring robots', *Body & Society*, 26(3): 31–60.

Emerson, R.M., Fretz, R.L. and Shaw, L.L. (1995) *Writing Ethnographic Field Notes*, Chicago, IL: University of Chicago Press.

Engelhart, K. (2021) 'What robots can—and can't—do for the old and lonely', *The New Yorker*, 31 May. Available from: https://www.newyorker.com/magazine/2021/05/31/what-robots-can-and-cant-do-for-the-old-and-lonely [Accessed 30 December 2021].

Jenkins, N. (2017) 'No substitute for human touch? Towards a critically posthumanist approach to dementia care', *Ageing & Society*, 37(7): 1484–1498.

Jenkins, N., Gorman, R., Douglas, C., Ashall, V., Ritchie, L. and Jack-Waugh, A. (2021) 'Multi-species dementia studies: Contours, contributions and controversies', *Journal of Aging Studies*, 59: 100975.

Koh, W.Q., Ang, F.X.H. and Casey, D. (2021) 'Impacts of low-cost robotic pets for older adults and people with dementia: Scoping review', *JMIR Rehabilitation and Assistive Technologies*, 8(1): e25340.

Koh, W.Q., Toomey, E., Flynn, A. and Casey, D. (2022) 'Determinants of implementing pet robots in nursing homes for dementia care', *BMC Geriatrics*, 22(1): 457.

Kramer, S.C., Friedmann, E. and Bernstein, P.L. (2009) 'Comparison of the effect of human interaction, animal-assisted therapy, and AIBO-assisted therapy on long-term care residents with dementia', *Anthrozoös*, 22(1): 43–57.

Marx, M.S., Cohen-Mansfield, J., Regier, N.G., Dakheel-Ali, M., Srihari, A. and Thein, K. (2010) 'The impact of different dog-related stimuli on engagement of persons with dementia', *American Journal of Alzheimer's Disease and Other Dementias*, 25(1): 37–45.

Minmin, L., Peng, L., Ping, Z., Mingyue, H., Haiyan, Z., Guichen, L., et al (2019) 'Pet robot intervention for people with dementia: A systematic review and meta-analysis of randomized controlled trials', *Psychiatry Research*, 271: 516–525.

Moyle, W., Jones, C.J., Murfield, J.E., Thalib, L., Beattie, E.R., Shum, D.K., et al (2017) 'Use of a robotic seal as a therapeutic tool to improve dementia symptoms: A cluster-randomized controlled trial', *Journal of the American Medical Directors Association*, 18(9): 766–773.

Nelson, R. and Westenskow, R. (2022) 'Evaluation of a robotic pet intervention protocol for older adults with dementia', *Canadian Journal of Recreation Therapy*, 1(1): 88–104.

Nolan, M.R., Davies, S., Brown, J., Keady, J. and Nolan, J. (2004) 'Beyond "person-centred" care: A new vision for gerontological nursing', *Journal of Clinical Nursing*, 13(s1): 45–53.

Rock, M.J. (2017) 'Who or what is "the public" in critical public health? Reflections on posthumanism and anthropological engagements with One Health', *Critical Public Health*, 27(3): 314–324.

Sharkey, A. and Wood, N. (2014) 'The Paro seal robot: Demeaning or enabling', in *Proceedings of Society for the Study of Artificial Intelligence and the Simulation of Behaviour (AISB)*, 40th Annual Convention held at Goldsmiths, University of London, 1–4 April 2014. Available from: http://www.doc.gold.ac.uk/aisb50/AISB50-S17/AISB50-S17-Sharkey-Paper.pdf [Accessed 13 March 2020].

Shibata, T., Wada, K., Saito, T. and Tanie, K. (2005) 'Human interactive robot for psychological enrichment and therapy', in *Proceedings of Society for the Study of Artificial Intelligence and the Simulation of Behaviour (AISB)*, Annual Convention held at University of Hertfordshire, April 2005, pp 98–109. Available from: https://citeseerx.ist.psu.edu/document?repid=rep1&type=pdf&doi=957b938c4a5e83dca32886ad358d8625574e6849#page=111 [Accessed 9 November 2022].

Shildrick, M. (2021) 'Queering dementia: Technologies, visceral prostheses and embodiment', *Lambda Nordica*, 26(2–3): 76–101.

Sparrow, R. (2002) 'The march of the robot dogs', *Ethics and Information Technology*, 4(4): 305–318.

Spradley, J.P. (1979) *The Ethnographic Interview*, New York, NY: Holt, Rinehart and Winston.

Stewart, A. (1998) *The Ethnographer's Method*, Thousand Oaks, CA: SAGE.

Technavio (2022) *Robotic Pet Dogs Market by Distribution Channel and Geography: Forecast and Analysis 2022–2026*. Available from: https://www.technavio.com/report/robotic-pet-dogs-market-industry-size-analysis [Accessed 11 January 2022].

Thodberg, K., Sørensen, L.U., Christensen, J.W., Poulsen, P.H., Houbak, B., Damgaard, V., et al (2016a) 'Therapeutic effects of dog visits in nursing homes for the elderly', *Psychogeriatrics*, 16(5): 289–297.

Thodberg, K., Sørensen, L.U., Videbech, P.B., Poulsen, P.H., Houbak, B., Damgaard, V., et al (2016b) 'Behavioral responses of nursing home residents to visits from a person with a dog, a robot seal or a toy cat', *Anthrozoös*, 29(1): 107–121.

Toohey, A.M. (2023) 'Considering cats, dogs, and contradictions: Pets and their relational influence on experiences of aging-in-place', *Canadian Journal on Aging*, 42(3): 506–515.

Toohey, A.M., Hewson, J.A., Adams, C.L. and Rock, M.J. (2017) 'When "places" include pets: Broadening the scope of relational approaches to promoting aging-in-place', *Journal of Sociology & Social Welfare*, 44(3): 119–146.

Valentí Soler, M., Agüera-Ortiz, L., Olazarán Rodríguez, J., Mendoza Rebolledo, C., Pérez Muñoz, A., Rodríguez Pérez, I., et al (2015) 'Social robots in advanced dementia', *Frontiers in Aging Neuroscience*, 7: 133.

Webb, J., Williams, V., Gall, M. and Dowling, S. (2020) 'Misfitting the research process: Shaping qualitative research "in the field" to fit people living with dementia', *International Journal of Qualitative Methods*, 19.

Zimolag, U. and Krupa, T. (2009) 'Pet ownership as a meaningful community occupation for people with serious mental illness', *American Journal of Occupational Therapy*, 63(2): 126–137.

9

Afterword: Towards an interdisciplinary approach?

Anna Jack-Waugh, Nicholas Jenkins and Louise Ritchie

As we were preparing this edited book, we learned of the death of Roger Payne in June 2023. News of his passing reminded us of his recordings of humpback whale song made during the 1960s and 1970s. His recordings introduced us to music that existed long before humanity and, in so doing, changed how these beautiful creatures were regarded around the world. His recordings demonstrated not only the existence of meaningful communication outside of the human species but also the beauty of this more-than-human singing, which reminds us of our place in a multi-species world: 'Whales and redwoods both make us feel small and I think that's an important experience for humans to have at the hands of nature. We need to recognize that we are not the stars of the show. We're just another pretty face, just one species among millions more' (Roger Payne, in White, 2016: 31).

Roger Payne's work led and influenced the preservation of whales and their environment, creating a wider impact on how humans perceived nature and conservation. Interestingly, such was his influence that the movie *Star Trek IV: The Voyage Home* featured humpback whales saving the world through their song. Now, over 50 years later, we hope that the voices contained within this edited book, diverse and polyphonic as they are, offer something of a new 'song' about dementia to that which we so often hear; an alternative to the one in which humanity is both the principal 'victim' and the primary 'saviour' in the global 'fight' against dementia. We humans, as Roger Payne so eloquently puts it, are not the stars of the show.

This has not been an easy book to prepare, and we cannot claim it is an exhaustive or definitive statement on the potential for multi-species approaches to change how we understand and respond to dementia. By inviting contributions from across the Multi-Species Dementia International Research Network and bringing these together, we have sought to stimulate thinking across disciplinary boundaries and borders about the ways in which this phenomenon, that we call dementia, may connect, entangle and bind us with other living beings and with the more-than-human world. In many respects, the chapters of the book represent a snapshot from across the network, which is itself an emergent and loosely affiliated collection of researchers and scholars from across disciplines, countries and continents, united by a shared interest in reaching beyond the 'human' in the search for new and less unconsciously anthropocentric ways of responding to dementia. We cannot claim to have ambitions on the scale of Roger Payne, and, for some readers, the chapters within this book may raise more questions than they provide answers. So, the question we wish to address briefly in this afterword is, 'What now?'

As we highlighted in our introduction to this book, one of our key aims as editors was to provide a foundation upon which a more truly interdisciplinary approach to multi-species dementia studies may be cultivated. Interdisciplinarity is a contested concept and means different things to different people, in different contexts. In practical terms, it involves combining methods and insights from two or more academic disciplines to accomplish a common task or achieve a shared objective. What is more contentious, however, is the level of integration – of knowledge, methods or ideas – that is to be achieved through interdisciplinary work. For some, it is sufficient simply that dialogue exists between different disciplinary knowledge, and integration is not required in order to further our understandings. For others, integration, or synthesis, is the goal of doing interdisciplinary work and success is to be measured through the extent to which new, and truly interdisciplinary, knowledge emerges from the collaboration.

In this book, we have brought together knowledge about dementia, that each seeks to explore our relations with different species, but which heralds from, at times, vastly different intellectual traditions. Chapters provided by Sordo (Chapter 3), and by Crilly et al (Chapter 4), for example, are rooted firmly in the scientific, (post)positivist tradition and provide state-of-the-art reviews on the nature of scientific understanding. These contrast starkly with chapters offered by Ashall (Chapter 6) and by Peel et al (Chapter 5), which provide reflexive and deeply personal accounts of their experiences of caring for and caring about aged canine companions. In contrast to Sordo, and to Crilly et al, their contributions sit firmly within anti-positivist, autoethnographic and (arguably) post-qualitative traditions. In between these two polarities, chapters prepared by Davies et al (Chapter 2), Toohey et al (Chapter 8), and by ourselves (Chapter 7) are rooted in the constructivist tradition yet retain key features of more 'traditional' approaches to qualitative inquiry. How, then, should we move forward towards a more interdisciplinary approach? Is it sufficient for these perspectives to sit alongside each other as polite, if somewhat distinct, intellectual bedfellows and companions? Should we, in contrast, seek to fuse the (post)positivist with the anti-positivist, the objective with the reflexive, and the multi-species with *multi-speciesism*, to produce a truly synthetic approach to exploring dementia within-and-across species lines? We wonder if such an approach would be possible, let alone desirable, given the differences in perspectives, knowledge and understanding that exists across these different contributions. And yet, arguably, it is not enough for these different perspectives to merely sit alongside each other, united solely by their inclusion of more than one species of biological (or, in the case of Toohey et al, non-biological) 'organism' within the scope of their inquiry. Little is to be gained by simply incorporating these different perspectives within, say, a single academic conference, a network, or an edited volume, without any attempt to interrogate their similarities and differences.

There is a potential third path towards interdisciplinarity that is neither defined by dialogue nor integration, namely, a *diffractive* approach. In the physical sciences, diffraction refers to the disruption of wave-based systems, in ways that create observable patterns of interference. As a metaphor, it provides a useful thinking tool in taking us towards what Haraway (1997: 16) refers to as 'another kind of critical consciousness … one committed to making a difference and not repeating the Sacred Image of the Same'. From a diffractive standpoint, difference is a central consideration. As Barad argues, by 'reading insights through one another' we become accustomed to 'attending to and responding to the details and specificities of relations of *difference* and how they matter' (Barad, 2007: 71; italics added). Thus, we believe, it is through a diffractive methodology that we can best develop an interdisciplinary approach to multi-species dementia research, scholarship, practice and policy making.

How, then, might we diffract insights about the behaviour of glial cells in animal brains (Sordo) or cytokines in human bodies (Crilly et al) with the experience of love, loss and personhood across species boundaries? This is an open question and one which we are just beginning to explore. The chapters in this volume, however, point towards several useful tools that we may use to create interference patterns that may, in turn, enable us to read insights from each other. Davies et al, for example, draw on the notion of *fabrication* to explore how scientific understandings of dementia are constructed and maintained within scientific communities. Within this framework, they argue that decisions about what and how to research are not only 'impregnated' by past decisions but are also 'impregnating' of future decisions. What, we wonder, may be possible within dementia science, if the knowledge of dementia in (non)human animals that Sordo reviews were to impregnate future decision-making. What might this multi-species form of fabrication look like? Might it, perhaps, lead to the involvement of animals as patients, or as (dare we say it) collaborators within dementia science? Might it lead to less reliance upon transgenic species of mice bred solely with dementia in mind – and for whom a life with neurocognitive disorder is a certainty – and towards a willingness to learn from animals who develop dementia organically as they age? Equally, we wonder how the *queer menageries* described by Peel et al might create new interference patterns in how we understand and respond to dementia. Queer menageries, as the authors highlight, refers to a 'political, experiential, and methodological approach to understanding the intersections of human and animal lives'. While Peel et al draw on this approach specifically to 'interrogate love and loss across species lines' the potentiality of this way of thinking to extend across the worlds of dementia is exciting. Indeed, *queer* appears in different parts of this book, as does the *posthuman*, referring both to non-heteronormative (multi-species) families as well as the potential to disrupt and make strange that which has been hitherto taken for granted. A multi-species approach to dementia is, we believe, *queering* because it makes anthropocentrism both visible and strange, and because it speaks to the experiences of many humans whose connections with animal *Others* have been ignored, mocked and belittled through both pronatalist and anthropocentric ideology. But what if these queer menageries extended beyond the family and into, for example, the laboratory, the care home or, even, the brain? Is it possible, for example, to understand relations involving *Toxoplasma gondii*, inflammation, *inflammaging* and dementia, that Crilly et al highlight in this volume, as queer menagerie formations? Might this way of thinking queer the 'battleground' approach to infection that is the dominant mode of attending within microbiology and, in so doing, offer new possibilities for understanding (micro) multi-species relationality in dementia? Related to this, and through our own chapter, we surface an ethic of *flourishing* that extends well beyond an ethic of '*Living Well*' or '*Living the Best Life Possible*' with dementia. How, we wonder, might *flourishing* serve to create interference patterns in, for example, how we understand 'infection' in dementia, as we affect a shift from a human-centric to a zōē-centric approach to preservation? These are speculative propositions, which we do not seek to address here. What they point to, however, is the potential for a *diffractive* interdisciplinarity to affect what matters in dementia, in both a material and semiotic sense. It is this potentiality, we argue, that an interdisciplinary, multi-species approach to dementia should attend to (*now*).

As we enhance our understanding of multi-species dementia, we also develop a more nuanced understanding of how to integrate a multi-species dementia approach in practice. In doing so, there is a need for a delicate balance between the rights of individuals, the welfare of animals and associated risks. For instance, careful consideration must be given to the rights and potential hazards faced by animals participating in assisted interventions within care facilities, as well as for the residents they interact with. Comprehensive guidelines are available, some of which include competencies and standards for practitioners, infection control measures and care environment management (RCN, 2019; SPAAI, 2021; 2024; Harrogate and District NHS Foundation Trust, 2023). There are critical differences in approaches in these guidelines. Some are precautionary, restrictive and wholly anthropocentric, and others, such as Association of

Animal Assisted Intervention Professionals guidelines, consider the needs of animals and humans with equity. None focuses on the specific needs of people with dementia and their families. Ensuring safe and beneficial multi-species dementia care practices requires the development of a comprehensive multi-species dementia practice guide. Such a resource would offer practical guidance on fostering collaborative working with animal-assisted intervention specialists, animal welfare, zoonotic disease management, the introduction of animals to individuals with dementia, and strategies for supporting families with pets in care settings.

While the perspectives of individuals living with dementia and their family caregivers are present throughout this text – illustrated, for instance, in Chapter 8, where family carers' viewpoints on the integration of robotic animals in care settings are showcased and our own work (Chapter 7) has been significantly shaped by the invaluable contributions of Anne Rankin, her late husband Henry, and their dementia assistance dog, Uno. However, we recognise that to advance the multi-species approach fully and its implementation in practice, we must move beyond conventional disciplinary boundaries and root our insights in the lived experiences of those living with dementia, their families, friends, practitioners and the animals involved. Embracing such a transdisciplinary approach enables academics to collaborate closely with individuals with lived experience and practitioners to tackle complex societal challenges.

The transdisciplinary approach is especially beneficial given the multifaceted policy and practical implications inherent in integrating a multi-species approach to dementia across society. These implications span from amplifying the voices of multi-species families navigating dementia, refining animal-assisted care practices, to facilitating meaningful engagement of individuals with dementia in research. This includes ensuring the availability of accessible information to facilitate informed decision-making regarding the involvement of animals in dementia research.

In concluding this book, it is important to note that the path towards a more multi-species understanding of dementia is fraught with potential pitfalls and controversies. As we have argued elsewhere (Jenkins et al, 2021), cultivating more multi-species approaches to dementia will inevitably involve engaging with sensitive, emotive and 'thorny' issues, including the use (or abuse) of animals in dementia research, as well as the application of concepts that have hitherto been reserved exclusively for humans – such as personhood, selfhood and rights – to members of other (non-human) species. Such issues have the potential to create strong fault lines and, if not well managed, to lead to accusations that multi-species perspectives are either indifferent to the plight of animals or, conversely, but the latest manifestation of 'woke science'. We hope that this emerging subfield of multi-species dementia studies may prove capable of navigating such controversies by cultivating a *science for the good* (Robbins, 2013) that is capable of working towards a way of 'being well together' (Kirk et al, 2019: 75) and doing so 'inside a world that is, however multiple, also shared, finite, and (in many ways) struggling' (van Dooren et al, 2016: 16).

References

AAAIP (Association of Animal Assisted Intervention Professionals) (2024) *Competencies for the Ethical Inclusion of Therapy and Facility Animals*. Available from: https://www.aaaiponline.org/assets/docs/AAAIPCompetencies.pdf [Accessed 29 March 2024].

Barad, K. (2007) *Meeting the Universe Halfway: Quantum Physics and the Entanglement of Matter and Meaning*, Durham, NC: Duke University Press.

Haraway, D. (1997) *Modest_Witness@Second_Millenium.FemaleMan Meets_OncoMouse*, New York, NY: Routledge.

Harrogate and District NHS Foundation Trust (2023) *Community IPC Policy for Care Home Settings. V3*. Available from: https://www.infectionpreventioncontrol.co.uk/wp-content/uploads/2019/07/CH-01-Animals-in-a-care-home-setting-April-2023-Version-3.00.pdf [Accessed 1 February 2024].

Jenkins, N., Gorman, R., Douglas, C., Ashall, V., Ritchie, L. and Jack-Waugh, A. (2021) 'Multi-species dementia studies: Contours, contributions and controversies', *Journal of Aging Studies*, 59: 100975, doi: 10.1016/j.jaging.2021.100975

Kirk, R., Pemberton, N. and Quick, T. (2019) 'Being well together? Promoting health and well-being through more than human collaboration and companionship', *Medical Humanities*, 45(1): 75–81.

RCN (Royal College of Nursing) (2019) *Working with Dogs in Health Care Settings*. Available from: https://www.rcn.org.uk/Professional-Development/publications/pub-007925 [Accessed 1 February 2024].

Robbins, J. (2013) 'Beyond the suffering subject: Toward an anthropology of the good', *Journal of the Royal Anthropological Institute*, 19(3): 447–462.

SPAAI (Standards of Practice for Animal-Assisted Interventions) (2021) Available from: https://therapyanimalstandards.org/downloads [Accessed 11 March 2024].

van Dooren, T., Kirksey, E. and Münster, U. (2016) 'Multispecies studies: Cultivating arts of attentiveness', *Environmental Humanities*, 8(1): 1–23.

White, J. (2016) *Talking on the Water: Conversations About Nature and Creativity*, San Antonio: Trinity University Press.

Index

References to figures appear in *italic* type; those in **bold** type refer to tables.
References to endnotes show both the page number and the note number (231n3).